의료상황영어

MEDICAL SITUATION ENGLISH

저자 김선옥

선문대학교

의료상황영어

초판 1쇄 인쇄 / 2015년 2월 25일
초판 1쇄 발행 / 2015년 2월 28일

지은이 / 김 선 옥
발행인 / 황 선 조
발행처 / 선문대학교 출판부
등록번호 / 제 9호
등록일 / 1998년 9월 25일
주소 / (336-708) 충남 아산시 탕정면 선문로 221번길 70
전화 / (041)530-2827　팩시밀리 (041)530-2979

디자인 · 인쇄 / 다해 (02)2266-9247

값　10,000원

ISBN 978-89-8423-768-1 93740

책머리에

우리 한국인은 초등학교부터 대학까지, 그리고 직장에 들어가서도 끊임없이 영어를 공부하고 있다. 일상생활 속에서 영어를 사용하기 위한 것이 목표가 아니고 평가를 위한 시험 위주의 영어공부를 하다 보니, 학교 영어시험이나 공인 영어시험에서는 고득점을 받아도 실제로 필요한 상황에서 영어를 제대로 구사할 수 있는 경우는 극히 드문 것이 사실이다.

이에 저자는 우리가 일상생활을 하면서 영어에 관심 있는 모든 사람들이 영어를 효율적으로 학습할 수 있는 방법과 어느 특정 분야의 전문가에 국한되지 않고 실제로 영어를 구사하는 데 있어서 누구나가 공감을 느끼는 영역이 무엇일까를 끊임없이 고민하던 중 <의료상황영어> 교재를 펴내게 되었다.

일상생활 속에서 누구나가 경험할 수 있는 기본적인 의료상황에서 구사할 수 있는 영어표현을 익히고 활용하는 데 본서의 목적이 있다. 부모, 자녀, 형제자매, 친척, 친구, 동료, 선배, 은사 등 주변의 누구나가 겪을 수 있는 통증 및 질병에 관해서 영어로 표현해 본다면 영어표현력이 훨씬 왕성해질 것이고, 또 더 오래 기억하게 되지 않을까 하는 것이 저자의 생각이다. 주변 사람들이 앓고 있는 질병 명을 영어로 찾아본다거나, 본인의 건강상 느끼는 변화를 영어로 생각해 보는 과정을 통해서 자연스런 영어 학습 및 활용을 유도하는 것이 저자의 의도이다.

본서는 표현 중심의 총 45개 단원으로 구성하였다. 매 단원은 Vocabulary Preview, Short Conversation, Pattern Practice, Useful Expressions 그리고 Vocabulary Review로 구성되어 있다. 한 학기 주당 3시간 3학점 강좌에서 1주에 3개 단원씩 다룰 것을 권한다.

원고를 집필하는 과정에서 끊임없는 격려로 저술방향에 박차를 가해 주신 단국대학교 영어과 김문수 박사님께 감사드린다. 아울러 글로벌시대 외국어교육의 중요성을 인식하여 올바른 학문의 길을 베푸는 선문대학교에 감사한다. 더욱이 이 책이 나오기까지 많은 관심과 심혈을 기울여 주신 선문대학교 출판부 관계자 여러분에게 감사의 뜻을 전하고 싶다. 마지막으로, 시간과 에너지가 많이 소요되는 저술과정에서 저자를 물심양면으로 지지해 준 가족들에게 머리 숙여 감사드린다.

2015년 2월

저자 김 선 옥

이 책의 특징

- 이 책은 45개 단원의 의료상황 영어 표현을 다루었다.

- Vocabulary Preview 항목에서는 그 단원에 나오는 의료상황 관련 어휘를 30개씩 정리 해 두었다. 의료상황 필수 어휘로 암기하여 활용한다면 영어표현을 자유롭게 구사하는 데 도움이 될 것이다.

- Short Conversation 항목에서는 제목 표현을 활용하여 일반적으로 주고받을 수 있는 A-B-A-B 형식의 짧은 대화를 엮어 놓았다. 각자의 상황을 고려하여 대화를 다양하게 엮어보는 연습을 한다면 표현력이 많이 향상될 것임을 확신한다.

- Pattern Practice 항목에서는 제목 표현 및 Useful Expressions 항목에 나오는 문장의 문형을 활용하여 패턴 연습을 할 수 있도록 하였다.

- Useful Expressions 항목에서는 제목 표현과 관련이 있는 기타 유용한 표현을 5개로 정리해 두었다. 제목 표현을 활용하여 Short Conversation을 작성한 것처럼, 여기에 나와 있는 각각의 표현을 이용하여 짧은 대화를 작성해 보는 연습을 한다면 영어표현력 향상에 많은 도움이 될 것이다.

- Vocabulary Review 항목에서는 기타 의료상황 영어 표현들을 통해 8개 내지 10개 정도의 어휘를 복습할 수 있도록 하였다.

CONTENTS

• 41 • 11. 얼마동안 깁스를 하고 다녀야해요?
How long do I have to wear this cast?

• 44 • 12. 부작용과 합병증에 주의하세요.
Beware of side effects and complications.

• 47 • 13. 심폐소생술은 배워두셨지요?
Are you trained in CPR?

• 50 • 14. 옷소매를 말아 올리세요.
Please roll up your sleeve.

• 53 • 15. 의사 선생님, 상처부위를 꿰매려고 하십니까?
Doctor, are you going to take stitches?

• 56 • 16. 교통사고로 목 부위에 부상을 입었어요.
I got a whiplash injury in an auto accident.

• 59 • 17. 저는 천식발작이 있어요.
I have attacks of asthma.

• 62 • 18. 저는 심장박동이 이따금 건너뛰어요.
Sometimes my heart skips beats.

• 65 • 19. 저는 어제 식중독에 걸렸어요.
I had food poisoning yesterday.

• 68 • 20. 저는 허리를 삐끗했어요.
I threw my back out.

• 71 • 21. 저는 손가락에 잔가시가 박혔어요.
I've got a splinter in my finger.

• 107 • 33. "하나, 둘, 셋!"하는 박자에 맞춰 구조팀원들이 환자를 몇 인치 들어 올렸어요.
On the count of three, the team members lifted the patient several inches.

• 110 • 34. 심폐소생술을 알아두면 언젠가는 곧 요긴하게 쓸 수 있을 거예요.
Your knowledge of CPR could come in handy any time soon.

• 113 • 35. 응급처치와 심폐소생술 강습을 받으셨어요?
Did you take First Aid and CPR classes?

• 116 • 36. 지혈대를 매는 방법을 아세요?
Do you know how to apply a tourniquet?

• 119 • 37. 어디가 불편하신가요?
What seems to be the problem?

• 122 • 38. 당신은 얼마동안 입원하신 거예요?
How long have you been hospitalized?

• 125 • 39. 대장암 가족력이 있습니까?
Do you have a family history of colon cancer?

• 128 • 40. 당신은 A형 간염에 대한 항체가 없어요.
You don't have an antibody for hepatitis A.

• 131 • 41. 나는 무릎관절에 문제가 있어요.
I have a problem in my knee joints.

• 134 • 42. 저는 매년 독감예방접종을 받아요.
I get a flu shot every year.

01
나는 숨이 차요.
I'm short of breath.

Vocabulary Preview 다음 단어의 뜻을 적어보세요.

❶ anemia ____________
❷ anesthetist ____________
❸ birth ____________
❹ blood cell ____________
❺ breath ____________
❻ cancer ____________
❼ chronically ____________
❽ collapse ____________
❾ condition ____________
❿ diagnose ____________
⓫ dizzy ____________
⓬ family doctor ____________
⓭ fuzzy ____________
⓮ hospitalize ____________
⓯ inflammation ____________
⓰ injury ____________
⓱ medicine ____________
⓲ metastasis ____________
⓳ midwife ____________
⓴ operation ____________
㉑ orthopedic ____________
㉒ pill ____________
㉓ radiotherapy ____________
㉔ recuperate ____________
㉕ recur ____________
㉖ recurrence ____________
㉗ registered ____________
㉘ shortage ____________
㉙ surgeon ____________
㉚ tzar ____________

Short Conversation

A: I'm short of breath.
나는 숨이 차요.

B: OK. Let's take a break.
좋아요. 좀 쉬도록 해요.

A: I get out of breath easily.
나는 쉽게 숨이 차요.

B: Let's exercise regularly to stay healthy.
건강을 유지하기 위해 규칙적으로 운동하기로 해요.

Pattern Practice

1 be short of + 명사

1. I am short of exercise.
2. They are short of orthopedic surgeons.
3. The hospital is short of 5 registered nurses.
4. Our country as a whole is short of family doctors.
5. Hospitals are short of medicines, blood and essential equipment.

2 have a shortage of + 명사

1. We have a shortage of doctors.
2. We have a shortage of midwives nationally.
3. We have a shortage of health professionals.
4. They have a shortage of trained health care staff.
5. The Army has a shortage of fully trained anesthetists.

Useful Expressions

1. Shall I have to be hospitalized?
저는 입원해야 될까요?

2 You have to recuperate at home.
댁에서 요양하도록 하세요.

3. Is it likely to recur? (= Is a recurrence likely?)
재발할 가능성이 있나요?

4. I feel dizzy.
현기증이 나요. (어지러워요.)

5. My head feels fuzzy.
머리가 멍해요.

Vocabulary Review 박스 안의 적당한 단어를 사용하여 빈칸을 채워보세요.

a. anemia	b. condition	c. dizzy	d. family doctor	e. midwives	f. operation
g. pill	h. recuperate	i. recurrence	j. shortage	k. surgeon	

❶ After an ___________, another serious inflammation recurred in his left knee.

❷ He needs more time to ___________ from his injury.

❸ He regularly gets checked for metastasis or a ___________ twice a year.

❹ I felt very ___________ all of a sudden and collapsed.

❺ ___________ play a crucial role in supporting normal birth.

❻ Take one ___________ three times a day.

❼ The blood is chronically short of red blood cells, a condition called _________.

❽ The cancer tsar himself admits that we have a ___________ of radiotherapy capacity in this country.

❾ The ___________ operated on my broken leg last week.

❿ Your ___________ can diagnose and prescribe medications for mental health issues.

02
외과수술로 치료될까요?
Will surgery cure it?

Vocabulary Preview 다음 단어의 뜻을 적어보세요.

❶ acne	________	⓰ fatal	________
❷ arthroplasty	________	⓱ injured	________
❸ back pain	________	⓲ insurance policy	________
❹ blood test	________	⓳ joint	________
❺ cancer	________	⓴ lump	________
❻ cast	________	㉑ medical	________
❼ come out	________	㉒ pill	________
❽ come round	________	㉓ relieve	________
❾ cough	________	㉔ removal	________
❿ diagnose	________	㉕ rescue	________
⓫ dislocate	________	㉖ sore throat	________
⓬ doctor	________	㉗ spread	________
⓭ ease	________	㉘ surgery	________
⓮ effect	________	㉙ upset	________
⓯ emergency	________	㉚ wart	________

Short Conversation

A: How's his leg?
그의 다리는 어때요?

B: Fortunately, his injury is not serious.
다행히도 부상이 심각하지는 않아요.

A: **Will surgery cure it?**
외과수술로 치료될까요?

B: Yes. And he will be discharged in a week.
예. 일주일 후에 퇴원할 거예요.

Pattern Practice

1 will + 타동사

1. This will help my upset stomach.
2. The medicine will have some effect.
3. These pills will help to ease the pain.
4. We will rescue those who are injured
5. This medicine will relieve you of your pain.

2 will + 자동사

1. His cancer will be fatal.
2. The surgery will be over soon.
3. The virus will spread to other people
4. The doctor will soon come round to see you.
5. The blood test results will come out next week.

Useful Expressions

1. I have a hard lump in my neck.
   나의 목에 단단한 혹이 있어요.

2. I broke my leg.
   나는 다리에 골절이에요.

3. I'm suffering from a back pain.
   나는 허리가 아파요.

4. I need a cast.
   나는 깁스를 해야겠어요.

5. I dislocated my right arm joint.
   나는 오른팔 관절이 탈골되었어요.

Vocabulary Review 박스 안의 적당한 단어를 사용하여 빈칸을 채워보세요.

a. acne	b. cast	c. dislocated	d. insurance	e. joint	f. lump
g. relieve	h. rescued	i. spread	j. surgery	k. upset	

❶ Arthroplasty is when an entire ___________ is rebuilt or replaced.

❷ He ___________ the boy at the risk of his own life.

❸ How did you cure your ___________?

❹ I don't want to ___________ my germs around the office.

❺ In a treatment room, another doctor put his leg in a ___________.

❻ Laser ___________ is used with the removal of warts.

❼ Many health ___________ policies cover ambulance rides for medical emergencies.

❽ She could feel a ___________ in her breast.

❾ The judoka ___________ his left shoulder during a competition last year.

❿ Use a humidifier to ___________ cough and sore throat.

03
어디 불편하신 거예요?
Don't you feel well?

Vocabulary Preview 다음 단어의 뜻을 적어보세요.

❶ ankle ________	⑯ overweight ________
❷ attack ________	⑰ pale ________
❸ bloodshot ________	⑱ pharmacist ________
❹ bring down ________	⑲ prescribe ________
❺ dizzy ________	⑳ prescription ________
❻ fall ________	㉑ sick ________
❼ fever ________	㉒ sick leave ________
❽ fill ________	㉓ sleep ________
❾ forehead ________	㉔ sleeping pill ________
❿ forty winks ________	㉕ sleepy ________
⓫ healthy ________	㉖ sprain ________
⓬ ice bag ________	㉗ tired ________
⓭ indigestion ________	㉘ weight ________
⓮ injured ________	㉙ well ________
⓯ lose ________	㉚ wrist ________

Short Conversation

A: Don't you feel well?
어디 불편하신 거예요?

B: I have a headache.
머리가 아파요.

A: I have some aspirin.
나한테 아스피린이 있어요.

B: I think I have indigestion.
아무래도 소화불량인 것 같아요.

Pattern Practice

1 Don't you feel + 형용사

1. Don't you feel dizzy?
2. Don't you feel better?
3. Don't you feel nauseated?
4. Don't you feel tired at all?
5. Don't you feel sleepy after lunch?

2 You don't look + 형용사

1. You don't look sick.
2. You don't look too pale.
3. You don't look overweight.
4. You don't look that healthy.
5. You don't look very well. Are you feeling okay?

Useful Expressions

1. How are you feeling today?
   오늘은 기분이 어떠세요?

2. You look quite pale.
   당신은 아주 창백해 보이네요.

3. Your eyes are bloodshot.
   당신은 눈이 충혈되어 있어요.

4. My stomach is upset.
   나는 배탈이 났어요.

5. I sprained my ankle.
   나는 발목을 삐었어요.

Vocabulary Review 박스 안의 적당한 단어를 사용하여 빈칸을 채워보세요.

a. bloodshot	b. fever	c. indigestion	d. overweight	e. prescription	f. sick
g. sick leave	h. sleeping pills	i. sleepy	j. sprained	k. well	

❶ Don't eat too fast, or you'll have an attack of ___________.

❷ He fell on the ice and ___________ his wrist.

❸ His eyes were ___________ from lack of sleep.

❹ I put an ice bag on her forehead to bring down the ___________.

❺ I was ___________ that day and missed the class.

❻ If you are sick or injured, you may take ___________ without pay for up to one year.

❼ I'm ___________, so I really want to lose weight.

❽ My doctor prescribed ___________ so I could get some sleep.

❾ She was so ___________ that she had forty winks in the afternoon.

❿ The pharmacist will fill your ___________.

04
어디가 불편하십니까?
What's the trouble with you?

Vocabulary Preview 다음 단어의 뜻을 적어보세요.

❶ adhesive bandage ______________
❷ blister ______________
❸ burn ______________
❹ chain smoker ______________
❺ chemotherapy ______________
❻ constipation ______________
❼ disorder ______________
❽ emergency ______________
❾ fatigue ______________
❿ fire drill ______________
⓫ fit ______________
⓬ headache ______________
⓭ heart disease ______________
⓮ hemorrhoids ______________
⓯ loose bowels ______________
⓰ occupational sickness ______________
⓱ potential ______________
⓲ rash ______________
⓳ relieve ______________
⓴ remedy ______________
㉑ ringing ______________
㉒ risk ______________
㉓ shingles ______________
㉔ side effect ______________
㉕ sneeze ______________
㉖ splitting ______________
㉗ surgery ______________
㉘ symptom ______________
㉙ viral infection ______________
㉚ weight ______________

Short Conversation

A: What's the trouble with you?
어디가 불편하십니까?

B: I have severe constipation.
변비가 심해요.

A: Did you take any medicine?
약을 드셔 보셨어요?

B: Yes, I did. But it didn't work.
예, 그런데 효과가 없어요.

Pattern Practice

1 What is + 단수 명사

1. What is a good remedy for a cold?
2. What is causing my morning sneezing fits?
3. What is the most common occupational sickness?
4. What is the latest news from the insurance company?
5. What is the worst part of wearing an adhesive bandage?

2 What are + 복수 명사

1. What are the symptoms of neck pain?
2. What are the risks involved with surgery?
3. What are the side effects of chemotherapy?
4. What are callers with emergencies advised to do?
5. What are the potential side effects of each treatment?

Useful Expressions

1. I have a headache.
   나는 두통이에요.

2. I have a splitting headache.
   나는 머리가 쪼개지는 것같이 아파요.

3. I have a stomachache.
   나는 복통이에요.

4. I have loose bowels.
   나는 설사해요.

5. My ears are ringing.
   귀에서 울리는 소리가 나요.

Vocabulary Review 박스 안의 적당한 단어를 사용하여 빈칸을 채워보세요.

a. burn	b. constipation	c. disorder	d. emergency	e. headache	f. heart
g. hemorrhoids	h. lose	i. rash	j. remedy	k. sleeping	

❶ Fiber-rich foods help relieve ___________.

❷ Good sleep is the best ___________ for fatigue.

❸ He has a hearing ___________, so you need to speak clearly.

❹ Her ___________ make sitting uncomfortable.

❺ I have trouble ___________ at night.

❻ In an ___________, call 911 for an ambulance.

❼ I've got a blister on my hand from a ___________.

❽ Shingles is a viral infection that causes a painful ___________.

❾ The chain smokers are at high risk for ___________ disease.

❿ What is the secret for those who successfully ___________ weight?

05
이것은 증세가 심각한 건가요?
Is this a serious case?

Vocabulary Preview 다음 단어의 뜻을 적어보세요.

1. acupuncture ________________
2. artificial respirator ________________
3. blood pressure ________________
4. breath ________________
5. burp ________________
6. chronic fatigue ________________
7. coma ________________
8. examination ________________
9. headache ________________
10. heart rate ________________
11. hurt ________________
12. lessen ________________
13. massive heart attack ________________
14. measure ________________
15. medical clinic ________________
16. migraine headache ________________
17. needle ________________
18. pharmacy ________________
19. prescription ________________
20. pulse ________________
21. reception desk ________________
22. scales ________________
23. serious ________________
24. sign in ________________
25. temperature ________________
26. thermometer ________________
27. thorough ________________
28. vital signs ________________
29. wash cloth ________________
30. weight ________________

Short Conversation

A: I feel extremely tired and sleepy all the time.
나는 항상 무척 피로를 느끼고 졸려요.

B: I think you have chronic fatigue syndrome.
당신은 만성피로증후군이에요.

A: **Is this a serious case?**
이것은 증세가 심각한 건가요?

B: Take it easy. Just try to get enough sleep every night.
안심하세요. 매일 밤 충분히 자도록 하세요.

Pattern Practice

1 Is this(지시 대명사) + 단수 명사(보어)

1. Is this an empty chair?
2. Is this drinkable water?
3. Is this your first time here?
4. Is this the way to the restroom?
5. Is this the right place to draw blood?

2 Is this(지시 형용사) + 단수 명사(주어)

1. Is this seat taken?
2. Is this man in a coma?
3. Is this wash cloth still cold?
4. Is this smell as bad as my burp?
5. Is this mattress too hard for you?

Useful Expressions

1. Take it easy. Nothing serious.
   안심하세요. 별것 아니에요.

2. I'll give you a thorough examination.
   세밀하게 진찰해보겠어요.

3. Have a good rest.
   푹 쉬세요.

4. Does it hurt when you move?
   움직이면 아프세요?

5. How long have you had this headache?
   두통은 언제부터 시작되었어요?

Vocabulary Review 박스 안의 적당한 단어를 사용하여 빈칸을 채워보세요.

a. acupuncture	b. burp	c. coma	d. hurt	e. pharmacy	f. prescription
g. pulse	h. reception desk	i. scales	j. thermometer		k. vital signs

❶ I thought ___________ would hurt, but I couldn't even feel the needles.

❷ I'll check your body weight. Please step on the ___________.

❸ Let me take your temperature. Please hold the ___________ under your tongue.

❹ Let's get your ___________--measure your blood pressure and your heart rate.

❺ My father had a massive heart attack then went into a ___________.
He is now on an artificial respirator.

❻ Take a deep breath and let it out slowly. I'll feel your ___________.

❼ The doctor wrote me a ___________ to help lessen my migraine headaches.

❽ The man is signing in at the ___________ of a medical clinic.

❾ You can get your medicine from the ___________.

❿ You have to say "excuse me" if you ___________.

06
의사선생님과 진료약속이 되어있어요?
Have you made an appointment with the doctor?

Vocabulary Preview 다음 단어의 뜻을 적어보세요.

❶ appointment	______	⑯ obese	______
❷ around the clock	______	⑰ overweight	______
❸ autism	______	⑱ patient	______
❹ blood test	______	⑲ physician	______
❺ cold	______	⑳ pregnant	______
❻ conceive	______	㉑ regularly	______
❼ cosmetic surgery	______	㉒ sick	______
❽ disposition	______	㉓ sneeze	______
❾ dropsy	______	㉔ sniffle	______
❿ fast	______	㉕ sue	______
⑪ genetic	______	㉖ swollen	______
⑫ injury	______	㉗ thirsty	______
⑬ malpractice	______	㉘ treat	______
⑭ medication	______	㉙ urine	______
⑮ nausea	______	㉚ vomiting	______

Short Conversation

A: I'm going to see the doctor now.
나는 지금 의사 선생님을 뵈러 갈 거예요.

B: **Have you made an appointment with the doctor?**
의사선생님과 진료약속이 되어있어요?

A: No, I haven't.
아니요, 되어있지 않아요.

B: I think you should make an appointment first.
예약 먼저 해야 할 거예요.
The doctor has a long waiting list of patients.
그 의사선생님은 대기환자수가 많아요.

Pattern Practice

1 Have you + p.p.(과거분사)

1. Have you heard about Dr. Schweitzer?
2. Have you been more thirsty than usual?
3. Have you managed to stick to your diet?
4. Have you conceived a child with any previous partners?
5. Have you experienced nausea or vomiting since the injury?

2 I have never + p.p.(과거분사)

1. I have never been pregnant.
2. I have never heard of autism.
3. I have never had any cosmetic surgery.
4. I have never been so sick in my whole life.
5. I have never smoked and have no genetic dispositions.

Useful Expressions

1. Now the doctor is engaged with another patient.
   지금 의사선생님은 다른 환자를 보고 계십니다.

2. The doctor has a long waiting list of patients.
   그 의사선생님은 대기환자수가 많아요.

3. Let me check your blood pressure.
   혈압을 재보겠습니다.

4. You need to take some laboratory tests.
   임상병리검사를 좀 해봐야겠어요.

5. The doctor is making rounds now.
   의사선생님은 회진중이에요.

Vocabulary Review 박스 안의 적당한 단어를 사용하여 빈칸을 채워보세요.

a. appointment	b. cold	c. cosmetic surgery	d. fast	e. injury	f. malpractice
g. medication	h. overweight	i. swollen	j. treats		k. urine

❶ Do you take any ___________ regularly?

❷ His legs were ___________ with dropsy.

❸ I have never been obese, but I was almost always ___________.

❹ I'd like to make an ___________ to see Dr. Kim.

❺ Now I feel a ___________ coming on with frequent sneezes and sniffles.

❻ Now, many young Korean men are choosing _________ to improve their looks.

❼ Please give me a ___________ sample in the cup.

❽ The physician was sued for ___________ after the patient died.

❾ The tiny hospital ____________ 1,500 people a day and is open nearly around the clock.

❿ You have to ___________ 12 hours prior to blood test.

07
저는 열이 있어요.
I have a fever.

Vocabulary Preview 다음 단어의 뜻을 적어보세요.

❶ acute	______	⓰ junk food	______
❷ affect	______	⓱ laryngitis	______
❸ bronchitis	______	⓲ phlegm	______
❹ chilly	______	⓳ pimple	______
❺ chronic	______	⓴ pneumonia	______
❻ constipation	______	㉑ runny nose	______
❼ contagious	______	㉒ scar	______
❽ cough	______	㉓ sore throat	______
❾ diabetes	______	㉔ stiff neck	______
❿ diarrhea	______	㉕ suffer from	______
⓫ face	______	㉖ swallow	______
⓬ high blood pressure	______	㉗ swelling	______
⓭ infection	______	㉘ tonsil	______
⓮ inflammation	______	㉙ tonsillitis	______
⓯ isolated	______	㉚ toothache	______

Short Conversation

A: I have a fever.
저는 열이 있어요.

B: Do you? Let me feel your forehead.
그래요? 이마에 열이 있나 볼게요.

A: I don't feel well. I feel chilly.
몸이 안 좋아요. 으슬으슬 추워요.

B: I think you have a cold. Take this medicine.
감기 걸린 것 같아요. 이 약을 드세요.

Pattern Practice

1 I have a + 증상

1. I have a cough.
2. I have a headache.
3. I have a toothache.
4. I have a stiff neck.
5. I have a runny nose.

2 I have + 질환/질병

1. I have diabetes.
2. I have diarrhea.
3. I have tonsillitis.
4. I have constipation.
5. I have high blood pressure.

Useful Expressions

1. Let me see your tongue and throat.
   혀와 목구멍을 보여주세요.

2. You have some swelling of your tonsils.
   당신은 편도선이 좀 부었어요.

3. I can't even swallow.
   저는 침을 삼킬 수도 없어요.

4. Face me and say, "Ah!".
   나를 향하여 “아!”해보세요.

5. I have a high fever and chills.
   저는 고열이 나고 으슬으슬 추어요.

Vocabulary Review 박스 안의 적당한 단어를 사용하여 빈칸을 채워보세요.

a. chronic	b. cold sweat	c. contagious	d. health	e. isolated	f. lungs
g. phlegm	h. pregnant	i. scar	j. swallow	k. voice	

❶ I always try to avoid things that will affect my ___________ negatively, such as smoking, drinking, and eating junk food.

❷ I have a hard, obstructive ___________ in my throat.

❸ I misused my ___________ and now I am suffering from laryngitis.

❹ It is hard to ___________ food because of my sore throat.

❺ People with ___________ diseases are isolated.

❻ Pneumonia is an infection or inflammation of the ___________.

❼ She's two months ___________, so she often has morning sickness.

❽ Unlike acute bronchitis, ___________ bronchitis is an ongoing, serious disease.

❾ When I woke up, my forehead and back were covered in ___________.

❿ You had better not pop the pimple. It'll leave a ___________.

08
주사 알레르기가 있나요?
Are you allergic to shots?

Vocabulary Preview 다음 단어의 뜻을 적어보세요.

❶ absorbent cotton ______________
❷ allergic ______________
❸ allergy ______________
❹ anesthetic ______________
❺ asthma ______________
❻ bloodstream ______________
❼ cell ______________
❽ corticosteroid ______________
❾ disease ______________
❿ dehydration ______________
⓫ flu ______________
⓬ giardia ______________
⓭ hay fever ______________
⓮ hive ______________
⓯ hospitalize ______________
⓰ infection ______________
⓱ inflammation ______________
⓲ injection ______________
⓳ I.V.(intravenous) drip ______________
⓴ medicine ______________
㉑ nasal spray ______________
㉒ nausea ______________
㉓ pollen ______________
㉔ prescribe ______________
㉕ rash ______________
㉖ rhinitis ______________
㉗ side effect ______________
㉘ sneeze ______________
㉙ surgery ______________
㉚ symptom ______________

Short Conversation

A: How may I help you?
무슨 일로 오셨어요?

B: I'm here to get the flu shot.
독감예방주사 맞으러 왔습니다.

A: **Are you allergic to shots?**
주사 알레르기가 있나요?

B: No, not that I know of. But I have an egg allergy.
아니요, 없습니다. 그런데 계란 알레르기가 있어요.

Pattern Practice

1 I am allergic to + 명사

1. I am allergic to fish.
2. I am allergic to cats.
3. I am allergic to shrimps.
4. I am allergic to peanuts.
5. I am allergic to shellfish.

2 I have an allergy to + 명사 (= I have a/an + 명사 + allergy)

1. I have an allergy to cats. (= I have a cat allergy.)
2. I have an allergy to pollen. (= I have a pollen allergy.)
3. I have an allergy to wheat. (= I have a wheat allergy.)
4. I have an allergy to avocados. (= I have an avocado allergy.)
5. I have an allergy to synthetics. (= I have a synthetic allergy.)

Useful Expressions

1. I'll give you a shot.
   주사 한 대 놓아드리겠어요.

2. I'll give you an insulin shot.
   인슐린주사를 한 대 놓아드리겠어요.

3. Press this absorbent cotton until the bleeding stops.
   출혈이 멈출 때까지 이 탈지면을 누르세요.

4. The nurse will put you on glucose drips.
   간호사가 포도당 링거주사를 놓아드릴 거예요.

5. You need an I.V. injection.
   링거주사를 맞아야겠어요.

Vocabulary Review 박스 안의 적당한 단어를 사용하여 빈칸을 채워보세요.

a. anesthetic	b. asthma	c. glucose	d. hay fever	e. hives	f. intravenous drip
g. medicine	h. relieve	i. rhinitis	j. side effect	k. sneeze	

❶ Cells use ____________ for energy after it moves into the bloodstream.

❷ Corticosteroids delivered as a nasal spray can reduce inflammation and control symptoms of allergic ____________.

❸ He has an allergy to cats that makes her ____________.

❹ In rare cases, giardia infection may cause a skin rash or ____________.

❺ ____________ is a common disease that effects the lungs.

❻ Nausea was a ____________ of the medication.

❼ He was hospitalized and given an ____________ after suffering dehydration.

❽ My family doctor prescribed a new ____________ for my nasal allergy.

❾ The patient was given an ____________ before surgery.

❿ The presence of pollen in the atmosphere causes ____________ in some people.

09
토할 것 같아요.
I feel like throwing up.

Vocabulary Preview 다음 단어의 뜻을 적어보세요.

❶ bitten	______	⓰ pepsin	______
❷ comfort stop	______	⓱ prevent	______
❸ contract	______	⓲ puke	______
❹ digestive enzyme	______	⓳ rasp	______
❺ digestive juice	______	⓴ soak	______
❻ encephalitis	______	㉑ sore throat	______
❼ fishbone	______	㉒ stethoscope	______
❽ gastric juice	______	㉓ stomach lining	______
❾ get carsick	______	㉔ stomachache	______
❿ get stuck	______	㉕ swallow	______
⓫ hiccup	______	㉖ throw up	______
⓬ hurt	______	㉗ tuberculosis	______
⓭ immunization	______	㉘ ulcer	______
⓮ measles	______	㉙ vomit	______
⓯ mosquito	______	㉚ vomit bag	______

Short Conversation

A: Can we have a comfort stop?
잠시 휴게소에 들렀다 갈 수 있어요?

B: Are you getting carsick?
차멀미하는 거예요?

A: **I feel like throwing up.**
토할 것 같아요.

B: You can use this vomit bag.
이 구토봉지를 사용하세요.

Pattern Practice

1 I feel like + 동명사

1. I feel like vomiting.
2. I feel like taking a long walk.
3. I feel like going out for dinner.
4. I feel like soaking in warm water.
5. I feel like having some ice cream.

2 I feel like + 문장

1. I feel like I'm getting old.
2. I feel like I have to puke.
3. I feel like I might throw up.
4. I feel like I am going to vomit.
5. I feel like I'm going to get sick.

Useful Expressions

1. Does it hurt when you swallow?
   침을 삼키면 아파요?

2. I can't hold food down.
   음식을 목구멍으로 넘길 수가 없어요.

3. I have a sore throat.
   목구멍이 아파요.

4. A fishbone got stuck in my throat.
   생선가시가 목구멍에 걸렸어요.

5. I hiccup a lot.
   딸꾹질이 많이 나요.

Vocabulary Review 박스 안의 적당한 단어를 사용하여 빈칸을 채워보세요.

a. ache	b. chest	c. die	d. gastric	e. immunization	f. mosquito
g. sore throat	h. stomach	i. swallow	j. tested	k. water	

❶ I exercised for a change, and now I ___________ all over.

❷ I have a terrible stomachache, I feel like I'm going to ___________.

❸ I was bitten by a ___________ and I contracted Japanese encephalitis.

❹ Measles can be prevented by ___________ at one year of age.

❺ My father has a ___________ and speaks with a rasp.

❻ Pepsin is a digestive enzyme found in ___________ juice.

❼ The doctor is listening to a patient's ___________ with a stethoscope.

❽ Ulcers occur when digestive juices burn a hole in the ___________ lining.

❾ You have ___________ negative for tuberculosis.

❿ You keep hiccuping. I think it'll stop if you drink some ___________.

10
약복용을 깜빡하고 거르셨어요?
Did you miss a dose?

Vocabulary Preview 다음 단어의 뜻을 적어보세요.

❶ apply ______	⓰ lump ______
❷ blood pressure ______	⓱ migraine ______
❸ boost ______	⓲ nausea ______
❹ cure ______	⓳ overdose ______
❺ directions ______	⓴ painkiller ______
❻ dosage ______	㉑ patient ______
❼ dose ______	㉒ pharmacy ______
❽ fill ______	㉓ physical ______
❾ get a facial ______	㉔ prescription ______
❿ hepatitis ______	㉕ prevention ______
⓫ immune system ______	㉖ scratch ______
⓬ infection ______	㉗ stomachache ______
⓭ jaundice ______	㉘ symptom ______
⓮ liver cancer ______	㉙ throbbing ______
⓯ liver disease ______	㉚ wear off ______

Short Conversation

A: **Did you miss a dose?**
약복용을 깜빡하고 거르셨어요?

B: Yes, I did. I forgot to take it this afternoon.
예, 오후에 복용하는 것을 깜빡했어요.

A: Missing one dose isn't going to cause much problem, but missing several doses is another story.
약복용을 한 번 거르는 것은 괜찮지만, 여러 번 거르게 되면 문제가 생길 수 있어요.

B: I'll keep that in mind. I'll take a dose regularly.
명심하겠습니다. 규칙적으로 복용하도록 하겠습니다.

Pattern Practice

1 Did you + 동사 원형

1. Did you sleep well last night?
2. Did you skip breakfast this morning?
3. Did you go to the doctor yesterday?
4. Did you take your blood pressure medication today?
5. Did you have any other symptoms with your stomachache?

2 When did you + 동사 원형

1. When did you break your leg?
2. When did you take your medicine?
3. When did you first notice the lump?
4. When did you have your last physical?
5. When did you get all the scratches on your face?

Useful Expressions

1. Please fill this prescription.
   여기 처방전을 가져왔으니 약을 지어주세요.

2. I have a prescription to be filled.
   여기 처방전을 가져왔어요.

3. Keep the dosage as directed.
   복용량을 지시대로 지키세요.

4. Overdose may prove harmful.
   과다복용은 해로울 수가 있어요.

5. Don't skip the dose.
   약복용을 거르지 마세요.

Vocabulary Review 박스 안의 적당한 단어를 사용하여 빈칸을 채워보세요.

a. cure	b. directions	c. dose	d. filled	e. head	f. hepatitis
g. hurt	h. produces	i. resist	j. skin	k. taking	

❶ A healthy diet should help your body ___________ infection.
❷ Apply the medicine after carefully reading the ___________.
❸ Did you know that your body ___________ vitamin D if you enjoy the sunshine?
❹ Jaundice is often seen in liver disease such as ___________ or liver cancer.
❺ Migraines usually involve a severe, throbbing pain on one side of the ___________, plus nausea.
❻ Prevention is better than ___________.
❼ The effects of the painkiller wore off, and my tooth began to ___________.
❽ The patient had her prescription ___________ at the pharmacy.
❾ You can boost your immune system by ___________ a bath.
❿ Your ___________ looks really clear and bright. Did you get a facial?

11
얼마동안 깁스를 하고 다녀야해요?
How long do I have to wear this cast?

Vocabulary Preview 다음 단어의 뜻을 적어보세요.

❶ antibiotic	______________	⓰ internal organ	______________
❷ blocked	______________	⓱ itchy	______________
❸ blood sugar	______________	⓲ large intestine	______________
❹ blow	______________	⓳ nasal cavity	______________
❺ braces	______________	⓴ physical	______________
❻ cast	______________	㉑ remedy	______________
❼ complication	______________	㉒ scratch	______________
❽ crooked teeth	______________	㉓ sinus	______________
❾ diabetes	______________	㉔ sinusitis	______________
❿ endoscopy	______________	㉕ slippery	______________
⓫ fatigue	______________	㉖ squeak	______________
⓬ feel numb	______________	㉗ straighten	______________
⓭ heal	______________	㉘ treatment	______________
⓮ hospitalize	______________	㉙ twist	______________
⓯ inflamed	______________	㉚ ultrasonography	______________

Short Conversation

A: How long do I have to wear this cast?
얼마동안 깁스를 하고 다녀야해요?

B: For about 6 weeks.
한 6주 정도요.

A: That long?
그렇게 오랫동안이요?

B: Yes. It takes time to heal.
예, 낫는데 시간이 걸려요.

Pattern Practice

1 How long do I have to + 동사 원형

1. How long do I have to wait?
2. How long do I have to be hospitalized?
3. How long do I have to keep from moving?
4. How long do I have to stay in the hospital?
5. How long do I have to take antibiotics for sinus treatment?

2 How often do I have to + 동사 원형

1. How often do I have to get a physical?
2. How often do I have to go see the doctor?
3. How often do I have to take the medicine?
4. How often do I have to monitor my blood sugar?
5. How often do I have to be monitored for diabetes complications?

Useful Expressions

1. I broke my leg.
   저는 다리가 부러졌어요.

2. I need a cast.
   저는 깁스를 해야겠어요.

3. I broke my left arm.
   저는 왼팔이 부러졌어요.

4. I twisted my right foot on a slippery rock.
   저는 미끄러운 바위에 오른발을 접질렸어요.

5. When can I expect to get the cast removed?
   저는 언제 깁스를 풀 수 있을까요?

Vocabulary Review 박스 안의 적당한 단어를 사용하여 빈칸을 채워보세요.

a. blow	b. braces	c. endoscopy	d. feel numb	e. gain	f. itchy
g. lose	h. nasal	i. remedy	j. rest	k. swallow	

❶ Good sleep is the best ___________ for fatigue.

❷ I don't feel very well, so I'll take a ___________ at home.

❸ I got an ultrasonography of my internal organs. I also got an ___________ of my stomach and my large intestine.

❹ I needed to wear ___________ to straighten my crooked teeth.

❺ I'm overweight. I want to ___________ some weight.

❻ It's so ___________ that I can't help scratching through my shirt.

❼ My legs ___________, so I can't walk.

❽ My throat hurts when I ___________ something.

❾ Sinusitis occurs when the ___________ cavity is blocked and becomes inflamed.

❿ When I ___________ my nose, my ears squeak.

12
부작용과 합병증에 주의하세요.
Beware of side effects and complications.

Vocabulary Preview 다음 단어의 뜻을 적어보세요.

❶ antibody ______
❷ bedsore ______
❸ breast milk ______
❹ breast feeding ______
❺ chronic ______
❻ complication ______
❼ contact dermatitis ______
❽ diabetes ______
❾ diarrhea ______
❿ fatality ______
⓫ food poisoning ______
⓬ injection ______
⓭ injury ______
⓮ intake ______
⓯ itchy ______
⓰ liver disease ______
⓱ medication ______
⓲ nausea ______
⓳ pregnancy ______
⓴ side effect ______
㉑ soothing ______
㉒ stem cell ______
㉓ stomachache ______
㉔ swine flu ______
㉕ swollen ______
㉖ symptom ______
㉗ therapist ______
㉘ therapy ______
㉙ treatment ______
㉚ withdrawal symptoms ______

Short Conversation

A: I have difficulty breathing.
저는 숨쉬기가 어려워요.

B: Did you follow your doctor's instructions?
의사 선생님 지시사항을 잘 지키셨어요?

A: I'm sorry. I smoked again. I'm suffering from withdrawal symptoms.
죄송합니다. 다시 담배를 피웠어요. 저는 금단 증상을 겪고 있어요.

B: **Beware of side effects and complications.**
부작용과 합병증에 주의하세요.

Pattern Practice

1 beware of + 명사

1. Beware of unproven therapies.
2. Beware of injury to tender parts.
3. Beware of swine flu conspiracy theories.
4. Beware of therapists who either push drugs immediately or dismiss drugs completely.
5. Beware of cheap jewellery containing nickel. It's the number-one cause of contact dermatitis, which leaves your skin red and itchy.

2 be aware of + 명사

1. Be aware of food poisoning.
2. Be aware of the dangers of too much vitamin intake.
3. Be aware of the fact that stem-cell injection treatments are illegal.
4. Be aware of the possible side effects associated with your medication.
5. Be aware of the following symptoms: stomach pain, nausea and vomiting.

Useful Expressions

1. Follow your doctor's instructions.
   의사의 지시에 따르세요.

2. This medication should not be used during pregnancy.
   이 약품은 임신 중에 복용을 금합니다.

3. This medication may appear in breast milk.
   이 약을 복용하면 모유에 나타날 수도 있어요.
   Consult your doctor before breast-feeding.
   수유하기 전에 의사와 상의하세요.

4. This medicine will give you a soothing sensation.
   이 약을 복용하면 증상이 완화될 거예요.

5. Don't share this drug with others.
   이 약을 다른 사람과 나눠먹지 마세요.

Vocabulary Review 박스 안의 적당한 단어를 사용하여 빈칸을 채워보세요.

a. bedsores	b. breast milk	c. fatality	d. injury	e. intake	f. itchy
g. soothing	h. symptoms	i. therapies	j. therapists	k. treatment	

❶ Antibodies found in ___________ protect babies against infection.
❷ Excessive sodium ___________ can cause health problems.
❸ He put a ___________ balm on his cut.
❹ If the ointments do not work, injections or other _____ need to be considered.
❺ Prompt ___________ can reduce your risk of complications.
❻ She dropped out of the race because of an ___________.
❼ The ___________ rate is much higher for patients with chronic liver disease or diabetes.
❽ The ___________ of food poisoning include stomachache, vomiting, and diarrhea.
❾ When a mosquito bites us, that spot gets ___________ and swollen.
❿ You have to reposition a patient frequently to prevent ___________.

13
심폐소생술은 배워두셨지요?
Are you trained in CPR?

Vocabulary Preview 다음 단어의 뜻을 적어보세요.

❶ administer ________	⓰ fall down ________
❷ ambulance ________	⓱ first aid ________
❸ appointment ________	⓲ healing ________
❹ available ________	⓳ infectious ________
❺ cold medicine ________	⓴ injured ________
❻ consultation ________	㉑ medical school ________
❼ CPR ________	㉒ melanoma ________
❽ dementia ________	㉓ over the counter ________
❾ dentist ________	㉔ paramedic ________
❿ determine ________	㉕ revive ________
⓫ diabetes ________	㉖ spot ________
⓬ drug ________	㉗ therapist ________
⓭ dying patient ________	㉘ trained ________
⓮ emergency number ________	㉙ treat ________
⓯ EMS ________	㉚ unconscious ________

Short Conversation

A: 911 Emergency Service. What is your emergency?
911 응급구조대입니다. 무엇을 도와드릴까요?

B: My friend is unconscious after falling down the stairs.
제 친구가 계단에서 넘어져서 의식을 잃었어요.

A: Our paramedics will be right over to help you.
우리 구급대원이 바로 도착할 것입니다.
Are you trained in CPR?
심폐소생술은 배워두셨지요?

B: Yes, I am. I will give him CPR.
예, 그에게 심폐소생술을 해보겠습니다.

Pattern Practice

1 be trained in + 명사

1. I am trained in first aid.
2. He is trained in dementia care.
3. She is trained in infectious diseases.
4. You are trained in how to treat this disease.
5. The therapist is trained in the art of healing.

2 be trained to + 동사

1. Everyone should be trained to use CPR.
2. I am trained to do this in medical school.
3. You are trained to determine the cause of death.
4. Paramedics are trained to administer certain drugs.
5. Your dentist is trained to spot melanomas that occur in your mouth.

Useful Expressions

1. Call for EMS(Emergency Medical Service).
   응급의료서비스를 부르세요.

2. Call 911 right away.
   즉시 119로 전화하세요.
   Call 911 for paramedics.
   119로 전화하여 구급대원을 부르세요.

3. Call for an ambulance,
   구급차를 부르세요.

4. There's an EMS vehicle coming.
   저기 응급의료서비스 차량이 오네요.

5. We are fighting to revive the dying patient.
   우리는 죽어가는 환자를 살리려고 안간힘을 쓰고 있어요.

Vocabulary Review 박스 안의 적당한 단어를 사용하여 빈칸을 채워보세요.

a. appointments	b. CPR	c. drug	d. EMS	e. infectious	f. injured
g. trained	h. over the counter	i. paramedics	j. revive	k. unconscious	

❶ Aspirin and cold medicine are available ____________.

❷ ____________ for consultations need to be made at least a day in advance.

❸ He attempted to ____________ his girl friend who had fainted.

❹ He learned how to do __________ in an emergency when he was ten years old.

❺ He was found lying ____________ on the road.

❻ It is an ____________ disease like the flu.

❼ People with diabetes must use this ____________ regularly.

❽ There were two people ____________ in the accident.

❾ We are well ____________ to handle any reasonable emergency.

❿ We called the emergency number and the ____________ were here in no time.

14
웃소매를 말아 올리세요.
Please roll up your sleeve

Vocabulary Preview 다음 단어의 뜻을 적어보세요.

❶ antibiotic ______	⑯ lack ______
❷ arteriosclerosis ______	⑰ LDL ______
❸ artery ______	⑱ litter ______
❹ blood flow ______	⑲ lower ______
❺ blood pressure ______	⑳ monounsaturated ______
❻ cholesterol level ______	㉑ nauseous ______
❼ cholesterol-rich ______	㉒ numb ______
❽ cigarette butt ______	㉓ prescribe ______
❾ circulation ______	㉔ roll up ______
❿ damage ______	㉕ shot ______
⓫ hardening ______	㉖ sputum ______
⓬ heart attack ______	㉗ temperature ______
⓭ hold out ______	㉘ urinate ______
⓮ irreversible ______	㉙ vital signs ______
⓯ keep an eye on ______	㉚ yawn ______

Short Conversation

A: I need to draw some blood from you.
채혈하겠습니다.
Please roll up your sleeve.
옷소매를 말아 올리세요.

B: Do I need to make a tight fist?
주먹을 꽉 쥐어야 하나요?

A: Yes, please. OK. Now you may relax.
예. 주먹을 쥐어 주세요. 됐습니다.
이제 주먹을 펴세요.

B: Are we done?
끝난 거예요?

Pattern Practice

1 Please + 동사원형

1. Please hold out your left arm.
2. Please let me check your vital signs.
3. Please collect some sputum in this cup.
4. Please check your name on the sticker.
5. Please take off your shoes and step on the scales.

2 Please don't + 동사원형

1. Please don't take a bath or shower today.
2. Please don't litter with your cigarette butts.
3. Please don't put too much stress on the knees.
4. Please don't take my lunch tray yet. I have not yet finished my lunch.
5. Please don't drive or operate heavy or complex machinery while taking this medication.

Useful Expressions

1. Let me check your blood pressure.
   혈압을 측정해보겠어요.

2. Let me take your temperature.
   체온을 재보겠습니다.

3. Watch your cholesterol count.
   콜레스테롤 수치에 유의하세요.

4. Shrimps are cholesterol-rich.
   새우는 콜레스테롤이 많이 포함되어있어요.

5. Are you nauseous?
   구역질이 납니까?

Vocabulary Review 박스 안의 적당한 단어를 사용하여 빈칸을 채워보세요.

a. blood flow	b. eye	c. hardening	d. monounsaturated	e. numb
f. prescribe	g. stress	h. urinating	i. yawning	

❶ Almost two thirds of the fat in avocados is ___________, a type that helps to lower levels of LDL or “bad” cholesterol in the blood.

❷ Are you keeping an ___________ on your cholesterol level?

❸ Let me give you a shot and ___________ some antibiotics.

❹ The lack of _______________ to your heart during a heart attack leads to irreversible damage to your heart muscle.

❺ The leg was going ___________ from lack of circulation.

❻ This process is called arteriosclerosis, or ___________ of the arteries.

❼ Urinate into the toilet a few seconds before ___________ in the sample cup.

❽ When ___________, try not to open your mouth too wide.

15
의사 선생님, 상처부위를 꿰매려고 하십니까?
Doctor, are you going to take stitches?

Vocabulary Preview 다음 단어의 뜻을 적어보세요.

❶ addiction ____________
❷ appointment ____________
❸ bleed ____________
❹ broken ____________
❺ cast ____________
❻ fat ____________
❼ forearm ____________
❽ gum ____________
❾ knit ____________
❿ laceration ____________
⓫ monounsaturated ____________
⓬ painful ____________
⓭ phobia ____________
⓮ plant ____________
⓯ plastic surgery ____________
⓰ polyunsaturated ____________
⓱ remove ____________
⓲ saturated ____________
⓳ scale ____________
⓴ scar ____________
㉑ sickness ____________
㉒ sterilize ____________
㉓ stitch ____________
㉔ suffer from ____________
㉕ suture ____________
㉖ take out ____________
㉗ tout ____________
㉘ treat ____________
㉙ trans fat ____________
㉚ withdrawal symptoms ____________

Short Conversation

A: You got a laceration on your head.
머리가 찢어지셨군요.

B: **Doctor, are you going to take stitches?**
의사 선생님, 상처부위를 꿰매려고 하십니까?

A: Yes, but the wound should be sterilized and dressed first.
예, 상처 소독과 치료를 한 후에요.

B: Make it soon. It is more painful.
빨리 해 주세요. 더 아파지는데요.

Pattern Practice

1 **Are you going to + 동사 원형**

1. Are you going to go see the doctor?
2. Are you going to go to the hospital?
3. Are you going to take your medicine?
4. Are you going to have plastic surgery?
5. Are you going to make an appointment?

2 **When are you going to + 동사 원형**

1. When are you going to go see the doctor?
2. When are you going to go to the hospital?
3. When are you going to take your medicine?
4. When are you going to have plastic surgery?
5. When are you going to make an appointment?

Useful Expressions

1. I put in five sutures.
   저는 다섯 바늘을 꿰맸어요.

2. I got a 5-cm laceration of my forearm.
   나는 팔뚝이 5cm나 찢어졌어요.

3. We'll take the stitches out next week.
   꿰맨 곳의 실밥을 다음 주에 뽑기로 해요.

4. Return in a week to have the sutures removed.
   일주일 후에 오셔서 꿰맨 곳의 실밥을 뽑으세요.

5. Will it form a scar?
   흉터가 생길까요?

Vocabulary Review 박스 안의 적당한 단어를 사용하여 빈칸을 채워보세요.

a. addiction	b. cast	c. dentist	d. gums	e. phobia
f. plants	g. scar	h. sickness	i. withdrawal	

❶ A few days after giving up smoking, I started to suffer from __________ symptoms.

❷ As she has a __________ of water, she doesn't swim.

❸ He had his broken arm in a __________ to help the bones knit together.

❹ He is now fighting his __________ to alcohol.

❺ Her cheeks became hollow after several days of __________.

❻ I went to the __________ and had my teeth scaled.

❼ Monounsaturated and polyunsaturated fats are generally found in __________ and are touted as healthy fats, unlike trans fats, saturated fats and cholesterol.

❽ My __________ bleed when I brush my teeth.

16
교통사고로 목 부위에 부상을 입었어요.
I got a whiplash injury in an auto accident.

Vocabulary Preview 다음 단어의 뜻을 적어보세요.

❶ bruise	________	⓰ mental illness	________
❷ burned	________	⓱ nosebleed	________
❸ chronic	________	⓲ overdose	________
❹ claustrophobia	________	⓳ physical exam	________
❺ closet	________	⓴ pill	________
❻ dentist	________	㉑ schizophrenia	________
❼ drunk	________	㉒ sciatica	________
❽ epilepsy	________	㉓ side	________
❾ esophageal spasm	________	㉔ splint	________
❿ food poisoning	________	㉕ stiff neck	________
⓫ get hurt	________	㉖ stiff shoulder	________
⓬ hand tremor	________	㉗ surgeon	________
⓭ hangover	________	㉘ swallowing	________
⓮ injured	________	㉙ take out	________
⓯ lump	________	㉚ whiplash injury	________

Short Conversation

A: What's wrong with your neck?
목이 왜 그래요?

B: **I got a whiplash injury in an auto accident.**
교통사고로 목 부위에 부상을 입었어요.

A: I hope it's not serious.
심각하지 않으면 좋겠어요.

B: Luckily, the injury is not serious.
다행스럽게도, 부상이 심각하지 않아요.

Pattern Practice

1 I got + 단수 명사

1. I got a lump on my head.
2. I got a bruise on my arm.
3. I got a nosebleed earlier today.
4. I got a physical exam at the hospital.
5. I got food poisoning in a Japanese restaurant.

2 I got + 형용사/과거분사

1. I got burned in the hand.
2. I got hurt below the knee.
3. I got injured by deep tackle.
4. I got sick when I drank some bad water.
5. I got drunk last night and now I have a hangover.

Useful Expressions

1. I got a bruise in an auto accident.
   교통사고로 타박상을 입었어요.

2. I have a stiff neck.
   목이 아파서 움직이지 못해요.

3. I have stiff shoulders.
   어깨가 아파서 움직이지 못해요.

4. I have a pain in my side.
   옆구리가 아파요.

5. I need to have my neck X-rayed.
   목 부위에 X-레이를 찍어야겠어요.
   I came here for an X-ray.
   저는 X-레이를 찍으러 왔어요.

Vocabulary Review 박스 안의 적당한 단어를 사용하여 빈칸을 채워보세요.

a. auto accident	b. claustrophobia	c. drive	d. mental	e. overdose
f. spasms	g. splints	h. teeth	i. tremor	

❶ His hands shook as though he had hand ___________.

❷ How many ___________ did the dentist take out?

❸ In some people, esophageal _______________ can lead to chronic swallowing problems and pain.

❹ Schizophrenia is one of the most common ___________ illnesses.

❺ She can't ___________ because she suffers from epilepsy.

❻ She gets ___________ in elevators and closets.

❼ Take one pill a day. Do not take an ___________.

❽ The surgeon set her broken arm in ___________ to hold it in position.

17
저는 천식발작이 있어요.
I have an attack of asthma.

Vocabulary Preview 다음 단어의 뜻을 적어보세요.

❶ accelerated ______
❷ angina ______
❸ anxiety ______
❹ appointment ______
❺ asthma ______
❻ attack ______
❼ breathe ______
❽ chest pain ______
❾ cough ______
❿ dizziness ______
⓫ draw ______
⓬ heart rate ______
⓭ heartburn ______
⓮ hypoglycemia ______
⓯ indigestion ______
⓰ inhaler ______
⓱ panic ______
⓲ pneumonia ______
⓳ prickly heat ______
⓴ sciatica ______
㉑ shortness of breath ______
㉒ spinning ______
㉓ strip ______
㉔ suffer from ______
㉕ sweating ______
㉖ symptom ______
㉗ trembling ______
㉘ tuberculosis ______
㉙ vertigo ______
㉚ wheeze ______

Short Conversation

A: I can't stop coughing.
기침이 멈추지 않아요.

B: Do you have a cold?
감기 걸렸어요?

A: **I have an attack of asthma.**
저는 천식발작이 있어요.

B: Do you need your inhaler?
흡입기 줄까요?

Pattern Practice

1 I have an attack of + 증상/병명

1. I have an attack of heartburn.
2. I have an attack of indigestion.
3. I have an attack of prickly heat.
4. I have an attack of tuberculosis.
5. I have an attack of hypoglycemia.

2 I have a/an + 증상/병명 + attack

1. I have a panic attack.
2. I have a angina attack.
3. I have an asthma attack.
4. I have an anxiety attack.
5. I have a pneumonia attack.

Useful Expressions

1. I feel blocked up in my chest.
   저는 가슴이 막힌 느낌이에요.

2. I feel short of breath when I walk a little.
   저는 조금만 걸어도 숨이 차요.

3. Please strip to the waist.
   허리까지 보이도록 상의를 벗으세요.

4. Take a deep breath, and let it lot.
   숨을 깊이 들이마셨다가 내쉬세요.
   Again, breathe in. Breathe out.
   다시 한 번 들이쉬고 내쉬세요.

5. Now turn around. Take a deep breath, and let it out.
   이제 돌아앉으셔서, 숨을 깊이 들이마셨다가 내쉬세요.

Vocabulary Review 박스 안의 적당한 단어를 사용하여 빈칸을 채워보세요.

a. appointment	b. breathing	c. draw	d. healthy	e. sciatica
f. stay away	g. strip	h. symptoms	i. vertigo	

❶ During an asthma attack, you may cough, wheeze and have trouble ________.

❷ I need to __________ some blood from you. Make a tight fist, please.

❸ I recommend that you __________ from irritating foods, alcohol and smoking.

❹ I suffer from __________ so it's hard for me to walk quickly.

❺ If you have frequent attacks of heartburn or indigestion, call your doctor for an __________.

❻ If you have _________ it seems as if the room is spinning around you.

❼ Some of the physical __________ include panic attack, dizziness, trembling, sweating, chest pain, accelerated heart rate, and shortness of breath.

❽ You seem to be very __________. Do you have any medical problems?

18
저는 심장박동이 이따금 건너뛰어요.
Sometimes my heart skips beats.

Vocabulary Preview 다음 단어의 뜻을 적어보세요.

❶ beat	________	⑯ irregular pulse	________
❷ Bell's palsy	________	⑰ paralyzed	________
❸ bowel movement	________	⑱ permanently	________
❹ cardiovascular	________	⑲ promote	________
❺ chronic asthma	________	⑳ pulse	________
❻ constipation	________	㉑ scab	________
❼ cramping	________	㉒ sensitive	________
❽ cupping	________	㉓ sharp pain	________
❾ dull pain	________	㉔ skip	________
❿ esophagus	________	㉕ spasm	________
⓫ fall asleep	________	㉖ spinning	________
⓬ go numb	________	㉗ stressed out	________
⓭ heart palpitations	________	㉘ take a break	________
⓮ hypertension	________	㉙ tuberculosis	________
⓯ insomnia	________	㉚ wound	________

Short Conversation

A: I think I'm getting heart palpitations.
제 심장이 몹시 두근거리고 있어요.

B: Why? Are you sensitive to caffeine?
왜요? 당신은 카페인에 민감하세요?

A: **Sometimes my heart skips beats.**
저는 심장박동이 이따금 건너뛰어요.

B: Did you see the doctor about your heart rate?
당신의 심박동수 문제로 의사 선생님께 진찰 받아보았어요?

Pattern Practice

1 Sometimes + 문장

1. Sometimes my hands go numb.
2. Sometimes my feet fall asleep.
3. Sometimes I get a pain around my heart.
4. Sometimes I have sharp pains in my stomach.
5. Sometimes I have terrible spasms in my esophagus.

2 문장 + sometimes

1. My bones ache sometimes.
2. My head is spinning sometimes.
3. I have to skip meals sometimes.
4. I need to take a break sometimes.
5. I feel exhausted and stressed out sometimes.

Useful Expressions

1. There's an occasional pause in my pulse.
   저는 맥박이 가끔 멈춰요.

2. I have a past history of tuberculosis.
   저는 폐결핵 병력(病歷)이 있어요.

3. I have chronic asthma.
   저는 만성천식이 있어요.

4. I have irregular pulses.
   저는 부정맥(不整脈)이 있어요.

5. I have a dull pain in my chest.
   저는 가슴이 뻐근해요.

Vocabulary Review 박스 안의 적당한 단어를 사용하여 빈칸을 채워보세요.

a. blister	b. brush	c. cardiovascular	d. constipation	e. cupping
f. paralyzed	g. pulse	h. scab	i. sleep	

❶ After her baby was born, she began ___________ therapy to cleanse her body.

❷ Fiber in the diet promotes regular bowel movements and helps avoid ___________ and cramping.

❸ Hypertension is one of the most common ____________ diseases in Asia, but many people know little or nothing about it.

❹ I burned myself on the stove and got a ___________.

❺ I sometimes lose a little bit of hair when I ___________ my hair.

❻ In his youth, he suffered an attack of Bell's palsy, permanently leaving the left side of his face partially ___________.

❼ Insomnia is the most common ___________ disorder.

❽ Until a ___________ forms over the wound, leave it alone.

19
저는 어제 식중독에 걸렸어요.
I had food poisoning yesterday.

Vocabulary Preview 다음 단어의 뜻을 적어보세요.

❶ abdomen	________	⓰ loose bowels	________
❷ appendicitis	________	⓱ organ	________
❸ appendix	________	⓲ pancreas	________
❹ bowel movement	________	⓳ pancreatic cancer	________
❺ brain tumor	________	⓴ rash	________
❻ coughing	________	㉑ remove	________
❼ crick	________	㉒ runny nose	________
❽ diagnose	________	㉓ stomach flu	________
❾ drop	________	㉔ surgery	________
❿ examine	________	㉕ symptom	________
⓫ eyesight	________	㉖ take out	________
⓬ flu	________	㉗ tonsil	________
⓭ headache	________	㉘ upset	________
⓮ hurt	________	㉙ weaken	________
⓯ immunity	________	㉚ wisdom tooth	________

Short Conversation

A: Why were you absent yesterday?
어제 왜 결석했어요?

B: **I had food poisoning yesterday.**
저는 어제 식중독에 걸렸어요.

A: I'm sorry to hear that. Are you feeling OK now?
안됐네요. 지금은 괜찮아요?

B: Much better than yesterday.
어제보다 훨씬 나아졌습니다.

Pattern Practice

1 I had + 명사

1. I had a runny nose.
2. I had really good eyesight.
3. I had a headache at school.
4. I had the flu for a couple of weeks.
5. I had a crick in my neck this morning.

2 I had + 명사 + p.p(과거분사)

1. I had my appendix removed.
2. I had my wisdom teeth pulled out.
3. I had my blood taken at a hospital.
4. I had my eyes examined yesterday.
5. I had my tonsils taken out last year.

Useful Expressions

1. I have the stomach flu.
   저는 배탈이 났어요.

2. I have rashes all over.
   저는 온몸에 두드러기가 났어요.

3. When's the last time you had a bowel movement?
   마지막으로 대변을 본 것이 언제였나요?

4. I have loose bowels.
   저는 설사를 해요.

5. Point with your finger where it hurts the most on your abdomen.
   당신의 복부에서 어디가 가장 아픈지 손가락으로 가리켜보세요.

Vocabulary Review 박스 안의 적당한 단어를 사용하여 빈칸을 채워보세요.

a. diagnose	b. getting rid	c. hospital	d. hurt	e. immunity
f. medicine	g. stomach	h. surgery	i. symptoms	

❶ A cold produces such ___________ as a headache, coughing, and a runny nose.

❷ Colon cleansing involves ___________ of the impacted fecal matter found in your intestines.

❸ He is recovering after the ___________ for a brain tumor.

❹ I'll give you some ___________ for the pain.

❺ It's better to avoid cold food when you have an upset ___________.

❻ She was taken to the ___________ with acute appendicitis.

❼ Since the pancreas, surrounded by other organs, is located deep in the abdomen, it is difficult to ___________ pancreatic cancer in its early stage of development.

❽ The level of ___________ is bound to drop when the body weakens.

20
저는 허리를 삐끗했어요.
I threw my back out.

Vocabulary Preview 다음 단어의 뜻을 적어보세요.

❶ ankle ____________	⑯ peritonitis ____________
❷ appendicitis ____________	⑰ polio ____________
❸ back pain ____________	⑱ scraped ____________
❹ broken ____________	⑲ sleep apnea ____________
❺ cirrhosis ____________	⑳ snoring ____________
❻ crippled ____________	㉑ sprain ____________
❼ Crohn's disease ____________	㉒ stomach ulcer ____________
❽ diverticulitis ____________	㉓ straighten ____________
❾ fall off ____________	㉔ strain ____________
❿ hairline fracture ____________	㉕ suffer from ____________
⑪ heart disease ____________	㉖ symptom ____________
⑫ kidney disease ____________	㉗ throw out ____________
⑬ medical condition ____________	㉘ twisted ____________
⑭ pancreatitis ____________	㉙ vegetarian ____________
⑮ pass out ____________	㉚ wrist ____________

Short Conversation

A: You look so painful. Are you OK?
많이 고통스러워 보여요. 괜찮아요?

B: **I threw my back out.**
저는 허리를 삐끗했어요.

A: Did you lift something heavy?
뭐 무거운 걸 들었나요?

B: No, I didn't. I took a false step down the stairs.
아니요, 층계를 내려가다가 발을 헛디뎠어요.

Pattern Practice

1 I 과거 동사 + my 신체 부위

1. I broke my arm.
2. I twisted my ankle.
3. I scraped my knee.
4. I strained my neck.
5. I sprained my wrist.

2 My 신체 부위 + is p.p.(과거 분사)

1. My arm is broken.
2. My ankle is twisted.
3. My knee is scraped.
4. My neck is strained.
5. My wrist is sprained.

Useful Expressions

1. I threw my back out when I took a false step down the stairs.
   저는 층계를 내려가다가 발을 헛디뎌서 허리를 삐끗했어요.

2. When I try to straighten my back, it hits me.
   허리를 피려고 하면 뜨끔해요.

3. I'm suffering from a back pain.
   저는 허리통증으로 고생해요.

4. I missed my step and sprained my ankle.
   저는 발을 잘못 디뎌서 발목을 삤어요.

5. I got a hairline fracture in my right ankle.
   저는 오른쪽 발목뼈에 금이 갔어요.

Vocabulary Review 박스 안의 적당한 단어를 사용하여 빈칸을 채워보세요.

a. broke	b. crippled	c. lost	d. lower	e. meat
f. medical	g. medicine	h. sleep apnea	i. twist	

❶ He was ___________ by polio as a child.

❷ I don't eat any ___________. I'm a vegetarian.

❸ I should take this ___________ for kidney disease.

❹ She fell off a ladder and ___________ her arm.

❺ She ___________ too much blood and passed out.

❻ Snoring may be a symptom of a more serious problem called ___________.

❼ The following _______________ conditions increase your risk of developing peritonitis: cirrhosis, appendicitis, Crohn's disease, stomach ulcers, diverticulitis and pancreatitis.

❽ Vegetarians usually have ___________ levels of heart disease.

21
저는 손가락에 잔가시가 박혔어요.
I've got a splinter in my finger.

Vocabulary Preview 다음 단어의 뜻을 적어보세요.

❶ bad cholesterol ______________
❷ bariatric surgery ______________
❸ blister ______________
❹ blood sugar ______________
❺ cavity ______________
❻ charley horse ______________
❼ cirrhosis ______________
❽ cold sore ______________
❾ corn ______________
❿ dermatitis ______________
⓫ eczema ______________
⓬ fingernail ______________
⓭ frostbite ______________
⓮ gastric bypass ______________
⓯ hearing aid ______________
⓰ inflammation ______________
⓱ injection ______________
⓲ insulin ______________
⓳ liver ______________
⓴ pins and needles ______________
㉑ rash ______________
㉒ remove ______________
㉓ saturated fat ______________
㉔ scorch ______________
㉕ splinter ______________
㉖ sty ______________
㉗ tear off ______________
㉘ tickle ______________
㉙ tinnitus ______________
㉚ tooth decay ______________

Short Conversation

A: I've got a splinter in my finger.
저는 손가락에 잔가시가 박혔어요.

B: Really? How did you hurt yourself?
그래요? 어쩌다가 그랬어요?

A: How do I take it out?
이걸 어떻게 빼죠?

B: Let me remove it from your finger for you.
제가 손톱에서 가시를 빼드릴게요.

Pattern Practice

1 I've got + 명사 + on

1. I've got a sty on my eye.
2. I've got a corn on my foot.
3. I've got a blister on my heel.
4. I've got a rash on my tongue.
5. I've got a cold sore on my lips.

2 I've got + 명사 + in

1. I've got a frog in my throat.
2. I've got a tickle in my throat.
3. I've got butterflies in my stomach.
4. I've got a charley horse in my leg.
5. I've got pins and needles in my leg.

Useful Expressions

1. I had my fingernail torn off.
   저는 손톱이 빠졌어요.

2. I ran a splinter into my middle finger.
   저는 가운데 손가락에 잔가시가 박혔어요.

3. I scorched my hand while cooking.
   저는 요리하다가 손을 데었어요.

4. I have frostbite on my right hand.
   저는 오른손이 동상에 걸렸어요.

5. I cut my hand with a razor.
   저는 면도날로 손을 베었어요.

Vocabulary Review 박스 안의 적당한 단어를 사용하여 빈칸을 채워보세요.

a. bariatric	b. blood	c. cirrhosis	d. diet	e. injections
f. skin	g. sugar	h. tinnitus	i. weight	

❶ Also called eczema, dermatitis is an inflammation of the ___________.

❷ Chocolate is not the cause of tooth decay. The ___________ in chocolate can cause cavities.

❸ Gastric bypass is the favored ___________ surgery in the United States.

❹ He had to give himself daily ___________ of insulin to help him control his blood sugar.

❺ Hearing aids are a common answer for the treatment of ___________.

❻ I'm on a ___________ now. I have to watch what I eat.

❼ In advanced ___________, the liver no longer works.

❽ Saturated fat can contribute to heart disease by increasing levels of bad cholesterol in the ___________.

22
나는 입맛이 없어요.
I have no appetite.

Vocabulary Preview 다음 단어의 뜻을 적어보세요.

❶ appetite	________	⓰ insurance	________
❷ blood sugar	________	⓱ intention	________
❸ burning	________	⓲ itching	________
❹ carpal tunnel	________	⓳ lack of sleep	________
❺ cavity	________	⓴ lie down	________
❻ colon cancer	________	㉑ medical care	________
❼ crutch	________	㉒ numbness	________
❽ dentist	________	㉓ osteoarthritis	________
❾ diabetes	________	㉔ palm	________
❿ diet	________	㉕ prevention	________
⓫ fat	________	㉖ rectal cancer	________
⓬ fiber	________	㉗ ruin	________
⓭ hair loss	________	㉘ scalp	________
⓮ heart disease	________	㉙ snacking	________
⓯ injection	________	㉚ tingling	________

Short Conversation

A: You are eating like a bird. Are you on a diet?
왜 그렇게 적게 먹어요? 다이어트 하는 거예요?

B: No, I'm not. **I have no appetite.**
아니요, **나는 입맛이 없어요.**

A: You look a bit tired. Are you OK?
당신은 약간 피곤해 보여요. 괜찮아요?

B: I'm OK. I think it's due to lack of sleep.
괜찮아요. 수면부족 때문인 것 같아요.

Pattern Practice

1 I have no + 단수 명사

1. I have no idea.
2. I have no feeling in my feet.
3. I have no dental or eye insurance.
4. I have no intention of quitting smoking.
5. I have no one to turn to but my older brother.

2 I have no + 복수 명사

1. I have no cavities.
2. I have no problems with my eyes.
3. I have no interests in becoming a doctor.
4. I have no health problems other than osteoarthritis.
5. I have no arms, but I can draw pictures with my toes and mouth.

Useful Expressions

1. How is your appetite?
   식욕은 어때요?

2. Please lie down a moment.
   잠깐 누워계셔요.

3. You need immediate medical care.
   곧 치료를 받으셔야 해요.

4. You should go on a strict diet.
   당신은 철저한 식이요법을 해야 돼요.

5. Watch what you eat.
   음식 조심하세요.

Vocabulary Review 박스 안의 적당한 단어를 사용하여 빈칸을 채워보세요.

a. appetite	b. cavity	c. crutches	d. dermatologist	e. diet
f. hand	g. history	h. insulin	i. scalp	

❶ A dentist checks and treats your teeth, and a ___________ is a skin doctor.

❷ Colon cancer and rectal cancer may be associated with a ___________ low in fiber and high in fat and calories.

❸ He broke his leg and is on ___________ now.

❹ He had to give himself daily injections of ___________ to help him control his blood sugar.

❺ In my family, we have a ___________ of heart disease and diabetes.

❻ Keeping your ___________ clean is vital for hair loss prevention.

❼ Snacking between meals ruins your ___________.

❽ The symptoms of carpal tunnel syndrome start slowly, and you may feel tingling, itching or burning feeling of numbness in fingers and the palms of the ___________.

23
저는 경련이 자주 나요.
I get charley horses often.

Vocabulary Preview 다음 단어의 뜻을 적어보세요.

❶ alleviate ______________
❷ anemia ______________
❸ beriberi ______________
❹ bleeding ______________
❺ bloated ______________
❻ blood poisoning ______________
❼ cancer ______________
❽ charley horse ______________
❾ chronic fatigue ______________
❿ cough ______________
⓫ cramp ______________
⓬ deficiency disease ______________
⓭ digest ______________
⓮ dizzy ______________
⓯ heredity ______________
⓰ leukemia ______________
⓱ limber up ______________
⓲ liver detoxification ______________
⓳ motion sickness ______________
⓴ pain ______________
㉑ relieve ______________
㉒ rickets ______________
㉓ salivary gland ______________
㉔ scurvy ______________
㉕ short of breath ______________
㉖ stomachache ______________
㉗ sweat ______________
㉘ throat ______________
㉙ toxin ______________
㉚ wound ______________

Short Conversation

A: Let's hit the road.
자, 출발합시다.

B: Wait a minute. I've got a cramp in my leg.
잠깐만요. 다리에 쥐가 났어요.

A: Are you OK? First, you should relax.
괜찮아요? 일단 긴장을 푸세요.

B: I'll be all right. I **get charley horses often.**
괜찮을 거예요. **저는 경련이 자주 나요.**

Pattern Practice

1 I get + 명사

1. I get enough sleep every night.
2. I get a stomachache when I don't eat.
3. I get a pain in my throat when I cough.
4. I get motion sickness every time I get in a car.
5. I get a sharp pain about an hour after I've eaten.

2 I get + 형용사

1. I get cold easily.
2. I get hot easily and sweat a lot.
3. I get short of breath when I walk.
4. I get dizzy sometimes after walking up the stairs.
5. I get bloated and can't seem to digest food properly.

Useful Expressions

1. I have pins and needles in my right leg.
   저는 오른쪽 다리가 따끔따끔 저려요.

2. I have sore feet from walking all day long.
   저는 온종일 걸었더니 발이 아파요.

3. Mentholatum can limber up tired muscles.
   멘소래담 로션을 바르면 피곤한 근육이 풀려요.

4. Take a warm shower to relieve leg cramps.
   다리경련을 풀어주려면 따스한 물로 샤워하세요.

5. I have cramps in my right leg.
   저는 오른쪽 다리에 쥐가 나요.

Vocabulary Review 박스 안의 적당한 단어를 사용하여 빈칸을 채워보세요.

a. anemia	b. blood	c. deficiency	d. dizzy	e. liver
f. relieve	g. role	h. toxins	i. untreated	

❶ After the wound was left ___________, blood poisoning developed.

❷ Chronic fatigue can be alleviated by ___________ detoxification.

❸ Did you know that your body releases 70 percent of its ___________ through breathing?

❹ Heredity also may play a ___________ in the development of salivary gland cancer.

❺ If you have severe bleeding, you could develop ___________.

❻ Leukemia, or cancer of the ___________, is the most common type in children.

❼ This medicine will ___________ you of your pain.

❽ Vitamins were discovered to correct ___________ diseases such as scurvy, beriberi, and rickets.

24
양쪽 뺨이 화끈거려요.
My cheeks burn.

Vocabulary Preview 다음 단어의 뜻을 적어보세요.

❶ asleep	________	⑯ itchy	________
❷ bloodshot	________	⑰ lining	________
❸ burn	________	⑱ overexposure	________
❹ cheek	________	⑲ puffy	________
❺ cramped	________	⑳ sandy	________
❻ dry eye syndrome	________	㉑ sinus trouble	________
❼ evaporation	________	㉒ skin cancer	________
❽ eye drops	________	㉓ smarting	________
❾ feverish	________	㉔ sore	________
❿ flushed	________	㉕ spinning	________
⓫ gastritis	________	㉖ stuffy	________
⓬ growling	________	㉗ swollen	________
⓭ hoarse	________	㉘ tear film	________
⓮ hot flash	________	㉙ ultraviolet rays	________
⓯ inflammation	________	㉚ watery	________

Short Conversation

A: My cheeks burn.
양쪽 뺨이 화끈거려요.

B: Your face is red. Are you feverish?
얼굴이 빨개요. 열이 있는 거예요?

A: I think so. I'm afraid I'm catching a cold.
예, 아무래도 감기 걸린 것 같아요.

B: Why don't you take the rest of the day off?
오늘은 일찍 가서 쉬는 게 어때요?

Pattern Practice

1 My + 신체부위(단수) + is

1. My nose is stuffy.
2. My face is flushed.
3. My head is spinning.
4. My neck is cramped.
5. My stomach is growling.

2 My + 신체부위(복수) + are

1. My legs are asleep.
2. My feet are swollen.
3. My knees are smarting.
4. My eyes are watery and itchy.
5. My arms are killing me from carrying all these bags.

Useful Expressions

1. I have a puffy face.
   얼굴이 푸석푸석하게 부어요.

2. I have hot flashes.
   얼굴이 화끈거려요.

3. This part of my head aches.
   이쪽 머리가 아파요.

4. My eyes feel sandy.
   저의 눈이 모래가 들어간 것 같은 느낌이에요.

5. I have sinus trouble.
   저는 부비강 질환이 있어요.

Vocabulary Review 박스 안의 적당한 단어를 사용하여 빈칸을 채워보세요.

a. blind	b. bloodshot	c. cold	d. eye	e. head
f. immune	g. skim	h. stomach	i. sunscreen	

❶ Dry eye syndrome is another ___________ disease caused by either decreased tear production or increased tear film evaporation.

❷ Experts recommend using a ___________ with an SPF of 30 or higher and say it is important to cover every part of your body that will be exposed to the sun.

❸ Gastritis is an inflammation of the lining of the ___________.

❹ My throat is not sore, but I'm a little hoarse from a ___________.

❺ Overexposure to ultraviolet rays can cause ___________ cancer.

❻ While I was suffering from pinkeye, I thought about the hardships of the ___________.

❼ Why are your eyes ___________? Here, try these eye drops.

❽ Your body has an ___________ system to fight off germs.

25
정식포장 약품으로 드릴까요, 일반포장 약품으로 드릴까요?
Brand-name drug or generic?

Vocabulary Preview 다음 단어의 뜻을 적어보세요.

❶ acupoint ______
❷ acupuncture ______
❸ anthelmintic ______
❹ antibiotic ______
❺ application ______
❻ blood pressure ______
❼ brand-name ______
❽ chicken pox ______
❾ digestive ______
❿ eradicate ______
⓫ expiration date ______
⓬ generic ______
⓭ go past ______
⓮ herbal ______
⓯ hyperhidrosis ______
⓰ make an appointment ______
⓱ malnutrition ______
⓲ measles ______
⓳ morning sickness ______
⓴ moxibustion ______
㉑ mumps ______
㉒ over the counter ______
㉓ painkiller ______
㉔ physical checkup ______
㉕ pimple ______
㉖ pregnant ______
㉗ prescription ______
㉘ pull out ______
㉙ vaccination ______
㉚ wisdom tooth ______

Short Conversation

A: I'd like to buy anthelmintic pills, please.
구충제 좀 주세요.

B: **Brand-name drug or generic?**
정식포장 약품으로 드릴까요, 일반포장 약품으로 드릴까요?

A: What's the difference?
차이가 뭔데요?

B: The generic pills are cheaper. They are the same except you don't have to pay for the name.
일반포장 약품이 좀 더 싸거든요. 브랜드 이름값을 지불하지 않을 뿐, 효능은 똑 같습니다.

Pattern Practice

1 Would you like to + 동사 원형

1. Would you like to see a doctor?
2. Would you like to get a physical checkup?
3. Would you like to reschedule your appointment?
4. Would you like to get your blood pressure checked?
5. Would you like to make an appointment with the doctor?

2 When would you like to + 동사 원형

1. When would you like to see a doctor?
2. When would you like to get a physical checkup?
3. When would you like to reschedule your appointment?
4. When would you like to get your blood pressure checked?
5. When would you like to make an appointment with the doctor?

Useful Expressions

1. Painkillers are prescription-only.
   진통제는 처방전이 있어야 판매가 가능해요.

2. Antibiotics are not sold over the counter.
   항생제는 처방전 없이 살 수 있어요.

3. This antibiotic is available by prescription.
   이 항생제는 처방전이 있어야 살 수 있어요.

4. Digestives and vitamin pills are over-the-counter drugs.
   소화제와 비타민제는 처방전 없이 살 수 있는 약이에요.

5. This medicine went past the expiration date.
   이 약품은 유통기한이 지났어요.

Vocabulary Review 박스 안의 적당한 단어를 사용하여 빈칸을 채워보세요.

a. bitten	b. digestive	c. heat	d. lack	e. pimples
f. pregnant	g. pulled out	h. sweats	i. vaccinations	

❶ Hyperhidrosis is a medical condition, where the body ___________ three- to four-times the normal amount.

❷ I can't get rid of the ___________ on my face.

❸ I got my wisdom teeth ___________ last year.

❹ Malnutrition is a medical condition, not just a ___________ of food.

❺ Many of the common childhood diseases such as measles, mumps, chicken pox were mostly eradicated with a national program of ___________.

❻ Moxibustion is the application of ___________ from an herbal bundle, used in conjunction with acupuncture, to stimulate the acupoints on the body and encourage self-healing.

❼ The part ___________ by an insect became swollen.

❽ When she was ___________, she often got morning sickness.

26
힘이 빠지세요?
Do you feel weak?

Vocabulary Preview 다음 단어의 뜻을 적어보세요.

❶ ailment ______	⑯ kink ______
❷ anemia ______	⑰ liver ______
❸ asthma ______	⑱ muscle ______
❹ bronchitis ______	⑲ nauseated ______
❺ chronic fatigue ______	⑳ panic disorder ______
❻ cirrhosis ______	㉑ parent ______
❼ dehydration ______	㉒ plastic surgery ______
❽ elderly ______	㉓ reflux esophagitis ______
❾ frequent ______	㉔ sick ______
❿ gastritis ______	㉕ smart ______
⓫ guilty ______	㉖ step out ______
⓬ health care ______	㉗ stretch ______
⓭ heartburn ______	㉘ symptom ______
⓮ illness ______	㉙ treatment ______
⓯ insurance ______	㉚ varicose vein ______

Short Conversation

A: Do you feel weak?
힘이 빠지세요?

B: Yes, I do. I have very low energy levels.
예, 기력이 너무 없어요.

A: Do you feel like you are always tired?
항상 피곤하다고 느끼세요?

B: Yes, I do. Am I suffering from chronic fatigue syndrome?
예, 제가 만성피로증후군인가요?

Pattern Practice

1 Do you feel + 형용사

1. Do you feel sick?
2. Do you feel good?
3. Do you feel nauseated?
4. Do you feel better now?
5. Do you feel guilty about lying?

2 How do you feel about + 명사/동명사

1. How do you feel about plastic surgery?
2. How do you feel about the rest of your body?
3. How do you feel about becoming a parent at 60?
4. How do you feel about getting treatment for your illness?
5. How do you feel about the Elderly Health Care Insurance?

Useful Expressions

1. Do you take alcohol?
   술 하세요?

2. I don't touch alcohol.
   술은 전혀 못해요.

3. Do you smoke?
   담배 하세요?

4. I just smoke socially.
   그저 사교상 빼끔담배를 해요.

5. What kind of food shall I avoid?
   저는 어떤 음식을 피해야 하나요?

Vocabulary Review 박스 안의 적당한 단어를 사용하여 빈칸을 채워보세요.

a. ailments	b. dehydration	c. illness	d. liver	e. muscles
f. smoke	g. step out	h. symptom	i. varicose veins	

❶ Frequent or constant heartburn is the most common ____________ of reflux esophagitis.

❷ Ginseng is prescribed alone or in combination with other herbs to treat chronic fatigue, anemia, gastritis, bronchitis, asthma and many other __________.

❸ If one drinks all his life, he may die of cirrhosis of the __________.

❹ Many women who work on their feet all day suffer from __________ and chronic leg and joint problems.

❺ My eyes smart with __________. Could you put out that cigar?

❻ People with severe panic disorder cannot drive or even __________ of the house.

❼ Stretch your arms to get the kinks out of your __________.

❽ Water is very important during and after a workout to prevent __________.

27
저는 당뇨병치료제를 복용해오고 있어요.
I've been taking antidiabetic pills.

Vocabulary Preview 다음 단어의 뜻을 적어보세요.

❶ antidiabetic ______	⓰ insulin shot ______
❷ appetite ______	⓱ migraine ______
❸ artificial sweetener ______	⓲ neurological ______
❹ blood pressure ______	⓳ operate ______
❺ boost ______	⓴ overweight ______
❻ chronic ______	㉑ pancreas ______
❼ colitis ______	㉒ recuperation ______
❽ colon ______	㉓ seizure ______
❾ constipated ______	㉔ sickness ______
❿ diabetes ______	㉕ sneeze ______
⓫ diagnose ______	㉖ stressed out ______
⓬ digestive disease ______	㉗ surgeon ______
⓭ disorder ______	㉘ symptom ______
⓮ epilepsy ______	㉙ tuberculosis ______
⓯ inflammation ______	㉚ urinate ______

Short Conversation

A: What seems to be the problem?
무슨 문제가 있으세요?

B: I'm urinating more frequently lately.
저는 최근에 화장실을 너무 자주 갑니다.

A: Are you taking any medication?
현재 복용중인 약이 있으세요?

B: **I've been taking antidiabetic pills.**
저는 당뇨병치료제를 복용해오고 있어요.

Pattern Practice

1 I have been + ~ing

1. I've been sneezing all morning.
2. I've been having trouble with my knee.
3. I've been exercising regularly to keep fit.
4. I've been taking medicine for my blood pressure.
5. I've been eating too much and not exercising enough.

2 I have been + p.p./일반 형용사/형용사구

1. I've been on a diet.
2. I've been constipated.
3. I've been stressed out.
4. I've been overweight all my life.
5. I've been in bed with a migraine all day.

Useful Expressions

1. Diabetes is usually controlled by insulin shots.
   당뇨병은 대개 인슐린주사로 조절이 돼요.

2. Insulin is produced by the pancreas.
   인슐린은 췌장에서 나와요.

3. When do I take this medicine?
   이 약은 언제 복용하죠?
   After meal and before retiring.
   식후와 취침 전에 하세요.

4. Take this medicine three times a day, 30 minutes after eating.
   이 약은 하루에 3회, 식후 30분에 복용하세요.

5. If that symptom continues or becomes severe, inform your doctor.
   그 증상이 지속되거나 심해지면 의사에게 통지하세요.

Vocabulary Review 박스 안의 적당한 단어를 사용하여 빈칸을 채워보세요.

a. appetites	b. colon	c. diagnosed	d. operated	e. scaled
f. seizures	g. sickness	h. stressed out	i. toothache	

❶ Colitis is a chronic digestive disease characterized by inflammation of the ___________

❷ Epilepsy is a common chronic neurological disorder characterized by ________.

❸ I can't chew any food well because of ___________.

❹ I have to get my teeth ___________.

❺ Laughter can speed up recuperation from ___________.

❻ Many doctors say that these artificial sweeteners can boost people's ___________, making them eat more.

❼ The doctor ___________ her case as tuberculosis.

❽ The surgeon ___________ on my broken leg last week.

28
이 약은 공복에 복용하지 마세요.
Don't take this medication on an empty stomach.

Vocabulary Preview 다음 단어의 뜻을 적어보세요.

❶ bronchitis ______
❷ catch a cold ______
❸ catch up on ______
❹ consult ______
❺ dizzy ______
❻ dose ______
❼ emphysema ______
❽ get a scar ______
❾ get worse ______
❿ grapefruit ______
⓫ internally ______
⓬ nauseous ______
⓭ overdose ______
⓮ persist ______
⓯ precautions ______
⓰ precedence ______
⓱ redness ______
⓲ resume ______
⓳ serious condition ______
⓴ shot ______
㉑ sign ______
㉒ skip ______
㉓ sleeping pill ______
㉔ stomach upset ______
㉕ swelling ______
㉖ symptom ______
㉗ terminal ______
㉘ treatment ______
㉙ unless ______
㉚ up the dose ______

Short Conversation

A: I feel nauseous and dizzy.
저는 메스껍고 어지러워요.

B: Did you miss a dose?
약 복용을 거르셨어요?

A: No, but I took some doses before meals.
아니요, 그런데 약 몇 번을 식사하기 전에 복용했어요.

B: **Don't take this medication on an empty stomach.**
이 약은 공복에 복용하지 마세요.

Pattern Practice

1 Don't take + 명사

1. Don't take this product internally.
2. Don't take this medicine before meals.
3. Don't take an overdose of sleeping pills.
4. Don't take a cold lightly. Go see a doctor.
5. Don't take your medicine with grapefruit juice.

2 What if I + 동사

1. What if I oversleep?
2. What if I get a scar?
3. What if I catch a cold?
4. What if I cut my fingers?
5. What if I lose my eye sight all of a sudden?

Useful Expressions

1. Take this medicine by mouth twice a day.
   이 약은 하루에 2회 경구투약하세요.

2. Take this medicine with meals to prevent stomach upset.
   위장장애가 없도록 이 약을 식사와 동시에 복용하세요.

3. What if I miss a dose?
   약복용을 깜빡 잊고 지나면 어떻게 하죠?

4. Don't double up the dose to catch up on the missed one.
   깜빡 잊고 지나간 복용량을 채우려고 복용량을 2배로 올리지 마세요.

5. Skip the missed dose and resume your dosing schedule.
   잊고 지나간 복용량은 거르고 원래의 복용스케줄을 따르세요.

Vocabulary Review 박스 안의 적당한 단어를 사용하여 빈칸을 채워보세요.

a. consult	b. directed	c. overdose	d. precautions	e. precedence
f. shot	g. skip	h. terminal	i. upped	

❶ Always read the ___________ on the bottle before using.

❷ Don't just take pills. Go to a hospital and get a ___________.

❸ Don't let it take ___________ over your health.

❹ Don't take this product unless ___________ by a doctor if you have a breathing problem such as emphysema or chronic bronchitis.

❺ He has ___________ cancer. With treatment, he may live another year.

❻ If pain persists or gets worse, if new symptoms occur, or if redness or swelling is present, ___________ a doctor because these could be signs of a serious condition.

❼ My doctor ___________ my dose because I didn't get better.

❽ Take one pill a day. Do not take an ___________.

29
당신은 응급처치나 심폐소생술을 할 수 있어요?
Can you administer first-aid or CPR?

Vocabulary Preview 다음 단어의 뜻을 적어보세요.

❶ administer ________	⓰ loss of consciousness ________
❷ clear the way ________	⓱ paramedic ________
❸ collapse ________	⓲ patient ________
❹ condition ________	⓳ perform ________
❺ contain ________	⓴ recommend ________
❻ CPR ________	㉑ remove ________
❼ cure ________	㉒ resuscitation ________
❽ decay ________	㉓ runny nose ________
❾ dentist ________	㉔ seizure ________
❿ disease ________	㉕ snore ________
⓫ filling ________	㉖ stagger ________
⓬ first-aid kit ________	㉗ stiff ________
⓭ headache ________	㉘ tartar ________
⓮ itch ________	㉙ unconscious ________
⓯ lidocaine ________	㉚ untreated ________

Short Conversation

A: Hey, look at the man in front of us.
어머, 우리 앞에 있는 저 남자 좀 보세요.

B: He is staggering. Oh, he collapsed.
그가 비틀거리며 걷고 있어요. 오, 그가 쓰러졌어요.

A: He looks unconscious. Let's call 911.
의식이 없는 것 같아요. 119에 전화합시다.

B: **Can you administer first-aid or CPR?**
당신은 응급처치나 심폐소생술을 할 수 있어요?

Pattern Practice

1 Can you + 동사 원형

1. Can you hear me all right?
2. Can you please clear the way?
3. Can you recommend a good dentist?
4. Can you do something about the itch?
5. Can you recommend a healthy diet that I can follow?

2 I can't + 동사 원형

1. I can't feel my toes.
2. I can't cure your disease.
3. I can't stand the cold weather.
4. I can't even move my neck properly.
5. I can't do anything because of my runny nose and headache.

Useful Expressions

1. Administer mouth-to-mouth resuscitation on the patient.
환자에게 구강 대 구강 소생술을 실시하세요.

2. I can give mouth-to-mouth resuscitation if necessary.
필요하다면 내가 구강 대 구강 소생술을 할 수 있어요.

3. Perform CPR on the patient before the paramedics arrive.
응급대원들이 도착하기 전에 환자에게 심폐소생술을 하세요.

4. The patient needs immediate help.
환자가 긴급한 도움이 필요해요.

5. Go ahead and bring me the first-aid kit.
응급처치 도구함을 어서 가져오세요.

Vocabulary Review 박스 안의 적당한 단어를 사용하여 빈칸을 채워보세요.

a. contains	b. cure	c. decay	d. feel	e. filling
f. snoring	g. stiff	h. untreated	i. wear	

❶ I can't read books because I can't see the letters. I think I need to _________ glasses.

❷ I can't sleep because my roommate is ___________ so loudly.

❸ I don't ___________ very well. Can you recommend a good doctor?

❹ If caffeine keeps you up at night, do not take this product in the evening since it ___________ natural caffeine.

❺ I'll give you some lidocaine, and then I'll begin working on this ___________.

❻ My neck is so ___________ that I can't even look back.

❼ Tartar is a hard yellowish substance that forms on your teeth and causes them to ___________ if it is not removed.

❽ These conditions require immediate care, because if left ___________, seizures and loss of consciousness can occur.

30
소변을 보기가 힘들어요?
Do you have any trouble urinating?

Vocabulary Preview 다음 단어의 뜻을 적어보세요.

❶ airsickness ______________
❷ allergy ______________
❸ Alzheimer's disease ______________
❹ bladder infection ______________
❺ breast cancer ______________
❻ bronchitis ______________
❼ burning pain ______________
❽ coma ______________
❾ complication ______________
❿ dehydration ______________
⓫ dementia ______________
⓬ diabetes ______________
⓭ diet pill ______________
⓮ dizziness ______________
⓯ family history ______________
⓰ health problem ______________
⓱ incurable disease ______________
⓲ intake ______________
⓳ pass water ______________
⓴ pneumonia ______________
㉑ pressure sore ______________
㉒ put on weight ______________
㉓ sore ______________
㉔ upset ______________
㉕ urge ______________
㉖ urinary frequency ______________
㉗ urinate ______________
㉘ urination ______________
㉙ urine ______________
㉚ yawn ______________

Short Conversation

A: Do you have any trouble urinating?
소변을 보기가 힘들어요?

B: No, I don't. But my urinary frequency has increased dramatically.
아니요, 그런데 배뇨빈도가 지나치게 심해졌어요.

A: How long have you had your symptom?
얼마나 그 증상이 지속되었나요?

B: For a couple of weeks. And I am unable to hold my urine once I feel the urge to urinate.
2주 정도 되었어요. 그리고 일단 소변을 보고 싶다고 느끼면 도저히 참고 있을 수가 없어요.

Pattern Practice

1 Do you have any + 단수 명사

1. Do you have any pain while urinating?
2. Do you have any history of severe headaches?
3. Do you have any airsickness medicine?
4. Do you have any medicine for an upset stomach?
5. Do you have any family history of breast cancer?

2 Do you have any + 복수 명사

1. Do you have any allergies?
2. Do you have any sores in your mouth?
3. Do you have any special health problems?
4. Do you have any family members with sleep problems?
5. Do you have any health conditions I should know about, such as shortness of breath or dizziness?

Useful Expressions

1. I have a burning pain on urination.
   소변을 보려면 뜨끔거리는 고통이 있어요.

2. Is your urine cloudy?
   소변색깔이 부옇게 나와요?

3. Is your urine cloudy or bloody?
   소변색깔이 부옇거나 피가 섞여 나와요?

4. Do you have to get up to pass water at night?
   밤에 소변을 보러 잠자리에서 일어나야 하나요?

5. Do you have any burning when you urinate?
   소변을 보려면 뜨끔거리나요?

Vocabulary Review 박스 안의 적당한 단어를 사용하여 빈칸을 채워보세요.

a. coma	b. dementia	c. head	d. incurable	e. intake
f. mouth	g. sore	h. urination	i. weight	

❶ Complications that may develop during a __________ include pressure sores, bladder infections and pneumonia.

❷ Do you have any aspirin? My __________ is killing me.

❸ He yawned without covering his __________.

❹ Smoking is the main cause of chronic bronchitis, which is an __________ disease.

❺ The most common form of __________ is Alzheimer's disease.

❻ Too much __________ of ice-cream made me put on fat.

❼ Untreated diabetes can cause dehydration by causing frequent __________.

❽ Using diet pills is not a safe way to lose __________.

31
환자를 들것위에 편안하게 눕히세요.
Lay the patient comfortably on the stretcher.

Vocabulary Preview 다음 단어의 뜻을 적어보세요.

❶ acid ____________	⑯ kidney stone ____________
❷ acidic food ____________	⑰ lung damage ____________
❸ anemia ____________	⑱ persistent ____________
❹ apply ____________	⑲ prescription ____________
❺ bed rest ____________	⑳ replace ____________
❻ blood transfusion ____________	㉑ rhinoplasty ____________
❼ cut back on ____________	㉒ safety strap ____________
❽ damaged tissue ____________	㉓ secondhand smoke ____________
❾ dialysis ____________	㉔ stomach pain ____________
❿ donor ____________	㉕ stretcher ____________
⓫ dosage ____________	㉖ surgery ____________
⓬ gout ____________	㉗ surgical repair ____________
⓭ heartburn ____________	㉘ treatment ____________
⓮ infection ____________	㉙ up the dosage ____________
⓯ intake ____________	㉚ weight-loss medication ____________

Short Conversation

A: How can we move the patient?
환자를 어떻게 옮기나요?

B: Lift the patient slowly. Be careful not to drop or injure him.
환자를 천천히 들어 올리세요. 환자를 떨어뜨리거나 부상을 입히지 않도록 조심하세요.

A: OK. What should we do next?
예, 알겠습니다. 다음엔 어떻게 하죠?

B: **Lay the patient comfortably on the stretcher.**
환자를 들것위에 편안하게 눕히세요.

Pattern Practice

1 You may need + 명사

1. You may need surgical repair.
2. You may need bed rest in the hospital.
3. You may need treatment for the rest of your life.
4. You may need dialysis until a suitable kidney donor is found.
5. You may need surgery to remove areas of persistent infection or repair lung damage.

2 You may need to + 동사

1. You may need to have damaged tissue replaced.
2. You may need to count calories and limit your salt intake.
3. You may need to stay in the hospital for one to two days.
4. You may need to take weight-loss medication for the rest of your life.
5. You may need to cut back on or avoid alcohol, caffeine or acidic foods.

Useful Expressions

1. Apply safety straps, and raise and secure the side rails.
   안전띠를 매어주고 측면 레일을 올려서 고정시키세요.

2. Roll the patient onto your upper arm and hold him against your chest.
   환자를 당신의 팔위에다 굴리듯이 올려서 당신의 가슴에 기대어 안으세요.

3. Do not lift or slide the patient onto the stretcher.
   환자를 들거나 밀어서 들것위에 올리지 마세요.

4. You may need one or two coworkers to lift the patient.
   환자를 들어 올리려면 1명이나 2명의 보조자가 필요할 수도 있어요.

5. Some patients may require a four-person lift.
   환자들 중에는 4명이 함께 들어 옮겨야 할 경우도 있어요.

Vocabulary Review 박스 안의 적당한 단어를 사용하여 빈칸을 채워보세요.

a. acid	b. anemia	c. intake	d. lung	e. medication
f. nose	g. patients	h. prescription	i. stretchers	

❶ At the time when the bones are growing, sufficient calcium ____________ is very important.

❷ Consuming a diet that is high in ___________ can result in heartburn, stomach pain, and more serious conditions like kidney stones and gout.

❸ If you have severe ___________ you may need to be hospitalized and receive blood transfusions.

❹ One type of plastic surgery is rhinoplasty, or ___________ surgery.

❺ Secondhand smoke is a known risk factor for ___________ cancer.

❻ The injured were carried away on ___________.

❼ The nurse was busy taking care of her ___________.

❽ You are not allowed to up the dosage without ___________.

32
환자를 들어서 이송하는 것은 환자의 건강에 지극히 중요해요.
Lifting and transporting a patient is vital for the patient's health.

Vocabulary Preview 다음 단어의 뜻을 적어보세요.

❶ administer ____________	⑯ ill ____________
❷ as directed ____________	⑰ intake ____________
❸ braces ____________	⑱ irregular ____________
❹ cardiac arrest ____________	⑲ lethargy ____________
❺ collapse ____________	⑳ life-saving ____________
❻ CPR ____________	㉑ overdose ____________
❼ daily dose ____________	㉒ prescription ____________
❽ depressed ____________	㉓ resuscitate ____________
❾ desperately ____________	㉔ scratch ____________
❿ dosage ____________	㉕ sit up ____________
⓫ emergency patient ____________	㉖ skip ____________
⓬ fast ____________	㉗ stretcher ____________
⓭ harmful ____________	㉘ supplement ____________
⓮ heart attack ____________	㉙ surgery ____________
⓯ hoist ____________	㉚ transfer ____________

Short Conversation

A: We should transfer the patient in a safe way.
우리는 환자를 안전하게 이송해야 해요.

B: What safety procedures should we take?
어떤 안전 수칙을 지켜야 하나요?

A: **Lifting and transporting a patient is vital for the patient's health.**
환자를 들어서 이송하는 것은 환자의 건강에 지극히 중요해요.

B: I see. Let's lift him slowly.
알겠어요. 그를 천천히 들어 올리죠.

Pattern Practice

1 You must + 동사 원형

1. You must stay in bed if you are ill.
2. You must ask your doctor for a prescription.
3. You must fast for 12 hours before this surgery.
4. You must stay in the hospital for another week.
5. You must eat healthy food and get plenty of exercise.

2 You must not + 동사 원형

1. You must not take aspirin.
2. You must not skip breakfast.
3. You must not drink if you drive.
4. You must not let yourself get depressed
5. You must not leave the house till your cold is quite cured.

32. 환자를 들어서 이송하는 것은 환자의 건강에 지극히 중요해요.
Lifting and transporting a patient is vital for the patient's health.

Useful Expressions

1. We tried every means possible to resuscitate the emergency patient.
   우리는 그 응급환자를 소생시키려고 온갖 수단을 동원했어요.

2. We tried desperately to resuscitate the heart attack patient.
   우리는 필사적으로 그 심장마비환자를 소생시키려고 애를 썼어요.

3. I followed all the life-saving procedures for the patient.
   나는 그 환자를 위해 모든 인명구조 절차를 따랐어요.

4. Remove watches and rings to avoid scratching the patient during transfer.
   이송도중에 환자에게 찰과상을 피하기 위하여 시계와 반지를 제거하세요.

5. When the patient collapses and is in cardiac arrest, you must administer CPR immediately.
   환자가 실신하거나 심장이 멈추었으면 즉시 심폐소생술을 시행해야 합니다.

Vocabulary Review 박스 안의 적당한 단어를 사용하여 빈칸을 채워보세요.

a. braces	b. climbing	c. directed	d. emergency	e. intake
f. resuscitated	g. stretcher	h. supplement	i. surgery	

❶ Her heart had stopped, but the doctors successfully __________ her.
❷ I have trouble __________ steps. I have to stop and catch my breath.
❸ Keep the dosage as __________. Overdose may prove harmful.
❹ The patient's lethargy after __________ is normal.
❺ Too much __________ of ice cream made me put on fat.
❻ Unable to stand or even sit up, he was hoisted onto a __________.
❼ Unless you eat plenty of fruits and vegetables, you may need to take a __________ of vitamin C to achieve the recommended daily dose of 1,000 milligrams.
❽ You have an irregular set of teeth. You need to have __________ fixed on your teeth.

33
"하나, 둘, 셋!"하는 박자에 맞춰 구조팀원들이 환자를 몇 인치 들어 올렸어요.
On the count of three, the team members lifted the patient several inches

Vocabulary Preview 다음 단어의 뜻을 적어보세요.

❶ abatement __________	⑯ motor tic __________
❷ Asperger's syndrome __________	⑰ nose twitching __________
❸ bipolar disorder __________	⑱ parallel __________
❹ bloodstream __________	⑲ Parkinson's disease __________
❺ cyclothymia __________	⑳ recovery __________
❻ diarrhea __________	㉑ relapse __________
❼ disease __________	㉒ relief __________
❽ disorder __________	㉓ rescue __________
❾ eye blinking __________	㉔ sensory deprivation __________
❿ fever __________	㉕ septicemia __________
⓫ grimace __________	㉖ shuffle __________
⓬ gurney __________	㉗ side effect __________
⓭ immunity __________	㉘ spoiled food __________
⓮ infection __________	㉙ stretcher __________
⓯ jerking __________	㉚ symptom __________

Short Conversation

A: The 911 rescue team arrived in the nick of time.
119구조팀이 때마침 아슬아슬하게 도착했어요.

B: Was the patient's life saved?
환자의 목숨을 살렸어요?

A: Yes, but they had difficulty moving the patient.
그들이 환자를 옮기는데 애를 먹었어요.
On the count of three, the team members lifted the patient several inches.
"하나, 둘, 셋!"하는 박자에 맞춰 구조팀원들이 환자를 몇 인치 들어 올렸어요.
She was finally rescued by the team.
결국 그녀는 구조팀에 의해 구조되었어요.

B: What a relief!
천만 다행이에요!

Pattern Practice

1 There is no + 단수 명사

1. There is no hope of his recovery.
2. There is no abatement in his fever.
3. There is no fear of a relapse of the fever.
4. There is no change in the patient's condition.
5. There is no way to acquire immunity to this disease.

2 There are no + 복수 명사

1. There are no bags under her eyes.
2. There are no risk free miracle drugs.
3. There are no medical facilities at all in that area.
4. There are no known side effects of sensory deprivation.
5. There are no medications to treat Asperger's syndrome.

Useful Expressions

1. Raise the bed to a comfortable working height.
   침대를 사용하기 편안한 높이로 올리세요.

2. Place the stretcher parallel to the bed, and lock the wheels.
   들것을 침대와 나란히 놓고 이동바퀴를 잠그세요.

3. Move the patient onto the stretcher, and slide your arms out from under him.
   응급환자를 들것에 옮기고 당신의 양팔을 그의 밑에서 슬그머니 빼내세요.

4. Push the gurney up to the second floor.
   바퀴달린 침대를 2층으로 밀고 올라가세요.

5. Lift or slide the patient onto the stretcher in a smooth, continuous motion.
   매끄럽고도 멈추지 않는 동작으로 환자를 들것에 밀어 올리세요.

Vocabulary Review 박스 안의 적당한 단어를 사용하여 빈칸을 채워보세요.

a. bipolar	b. bloodstream	c. diarrhea	d. fever	e. grimacing
f. motor tics	g. recovery	h. sick	i. treatments	

❶ Cyclothymia is a mild form of ___________ disorder.

❷ He has increasingly shown symptoms of Parkinson's, as shuffling his feet and sometimes ___________ in pain.

❸ I felt her forehead, and she had a ___________.

❹ I had some spoiled food and had ___________ all night.

❺ Septicemia can happen when an infection in the body enters the __________.

❻ She's never been absent before. Maybe she's ___________.

❼ Simple _____________ can be explained as eye blinking, nose twitching, and rapid jerking of any part of the body.

❽ What ___________ do you recommend for this disorder?

33. "하나, 둘, 셋!"하는 박자에 맞춰 구조팀원들이 환자를 몇 인치 들어 올렸어요.
On the count of three, the team members lifted the patient several inches.

34
심폐소생술을 알아두면 언젠가는 곧 요긴하게 쓸 수 있을 거예요.
Your knowledge of CPR could come in handy any time soon.

Vocabulary Preview 다음 단어의 뜻을 적어보세요.

❶ Adam's apple	______	⓰ nutritious	______
❷ airway	______	⓱ organ	______
❸ apply	______	⓲ oxygen	______
❹ Bell's palsy	______	⓳ paralysis	______
❺ bladder	______	⓴ perform CPR	______
❻ blinking	______	㉑ picky eater	______
❼ breathing	______	㉒ pump the blood	______
❽ chest compression	______	㉓ rescue breath	______
❾ come in handy	______	㉔ skinny	______
❿ cystitis	______	㉕ smell sour	______
⓫ dizzy	______	㉖ soften	______
⓬ exposed	______	㉗ supply	______
⓭ facial tic	______	㉘ tip	______
⓮ inflammation	______	㉙ twitching	______
⓯ medical term	______	㉚ weight	______

Short Conversation

A: Do you know how to administer CPR?
심폐소생술 할 줄 알아요?

B: No, I don't. But I know I should learn how to perform CPR.
아니요, 그런데 제가 심폐소생술을 배워야 한다는 것은 알아요.

A: **Your knowledge of CPR could come in handy any time soon.**
심폐소생술을 알아두면 언젠가는 곧 요긴하게 쓸 수 있을 거예요.

B: I'm not sure I can do it, but can you tell me how to give CPR?
제가 할 수 있을지는 모르겠지만, 저에게 심폐소생술 방법을 알려주시겠어요?

Pattern Practice

1 You should + 동사 원형

1. You should go see a doctor.
2. You should be at home resting.
3. You should alarm yourself when your heart is hurting.
4. You should eat nutritious meals to keep yourself healthy.
5. You should take pills three times a day within 30 minutes after meals.

2 You should not + 동사 원형

1. You should not be a picky eater.
2. You should not drink milk if it smells sour.
3. You should not eat too much. Watch your weight.
4. You should not exercise if you are dizzy and sleepy.
5. You should not do too much exercise before you go to bed.

34. 심폐소생술을 알아두면 언젠가는 곧 요긴하게 쓸 수 있을 거예요.
Your knowledge of CPR could come in handy any time soon.

Useful Expressions

1. Check for breathing before you perform CPR.
   심폐소생술을 실시하기 전에 호흡이 있는지를 확인하세요.

2. Start chest compressions and give rescue breaths.
   흉부압박을 시작하고 구조호흡을 제공하세요.

3. This is where you should begin your compressions.
   여기가 바로 흉부압박을 가하는 곳입니다.

4. The guidelines for CPR are 30 chest compressions to two breaths.
   호흡 2회에 흉부압박 30회를 가하는 것이 심폐소생술의 가이드라인입니다.

5. The compressions will continue pumping the blood to all organs, while the breaths supply the blood with oxygen.
   압박동작으로 혈액이 지속적으로 모든 장기로 퍼져 들어가면서,
   호흡이 혈액에 산소를 공급합니다.

Vocabulary Review 박스 안의 적당한 단어를 사용하여 빈칸을 채워보세요.

a. Adam's apple	b. bladder	c. blood	d. facial tic	e. paralysis
f. put on	g. rest	h. smoking	i. soften	

❶ An example of a ___________ is mouth twitching or rapidly blinking eyes.
❷ Apply this lotion on your hands. It will ___________ your skin.
❸ Bell's palsy causes sudden weakness and ___________ in your facial muscles.
❹ Cystitis is the medical term for inflammation of the ___________.
❺ Gently tip his head back so that the ___________ is exposed to clear his airways and open his mouth.
❻ It will be all over with your health if you keep on ___________.
❼ You should ___________ some weight. You look a little too skinny.
❽ You should ___________ if you're tired.

35

응급처치와 심폐소생술 강습을 받으셨어요?
Did you take First Aid and CPR classes?

Vocabulary Preview 다음 단어의 뜻을 적어보세요.

❶ acne scar ______________
❷ alopecia ______________
❸ Band-Aid ______________
❹ bloated ______________
❺ bruise ______________
❻ bump ______________
❼ bumpy ______________
❽ CPR-smart ______________
❾ degenerative ______________
❿ drowned ______________
⓫ emergency ______________
⓬ eye blinking ______________
⓭ facial tic ______________
⓮ hair loss ______________
⓯ indigestion ______________
⓰ kiss of life ______________
⓱ life-saving ______________
⓲ medical term ______________
⓳ nervous system ______________
⓴ nursing ______________
㉑ overuse ______________
㉒ paralysis ______________
㉓ Parkinson's disease ______________
㉔ potentially ______________
㉕ scratch ______________
㉖ split ______________
㉗ substantia nigra ______________
㉘ swollen ______________
㉙ Tourette's syndrome ______________
㉚ vocal cords ______________

Short Conversation

A: **Did you take First Aid and CPR classes?**
응급처치와 심폐소생술 강습을 받으셨어요?

B: I took a CPR class last month.
예, 나는 지난달에 심폐소생술 강습을 받았어요.

A: Did you get your CPR certification?
심폐소생술 자격증을 받았어요?

B: Yes, did. I'm taking a First Aid training class now.
예, 지금은 응급처치훈련 강습을 받고 있어요.

Pattern Practice

1 How did you + 동사 원형

1. How did you split your lip?
2. How did you cure your acne?
3. How did you bruise your arm?
4. How did you get that bump on your forehead?
5. How did you come by that scratch on your cheek?

2 Why did you + 동사 원형

1. Why did you stay up late?
2. Why did you drink so much?
3. Why did you ask me about drugs?
4. Why did you decide to go into nursing?
5. Why did you have a Band-Aid on your face?

Useful Expressions

1. I received certified CPR training last month.
   나는 지난달에 심폐소생술 공인과정 훈련을 받았어요.

2. CPR is a potentially life-saving procedure for everyone.
   심폐소생술은 누구에게나 잠재적으로 생명을 구할 수 있는 절차입니다.

3. CPR is used to bring back someone who has stopped breathing.
   심폐소생술은 호흡을 멈춘 사람을 소생시키기 위해 사용됩니다.

4. Everyone is encouraged to prevent, prepare for and respond to emergencies.
   누구나 응급상황을 예방하고 대비하며 즉각 대응하는 것이 좋습니다.

5. A CPR-smart lady gave a kiss of life to her drowned daughter.
   심폐소생술을 잘 아는 여인이 익사한 자기 딸에게 구강 대 구강 소생술을 시행했어요.

Vocabulary Review 박스 안의 적당한 단어를 사용하여 빈칸을 채워보세요.

a. bloated	b. bruised	c. bumpy	d. degenerative	e. doctor
f. facial tic	g. hair loss	h. split	i. swollen	

❶ Alopecia is the general medical term for ___________.

❷ His face is ___________ because of the acne scars.

❸ I have indigestion, and my stomach feels ___________.

❹ I have my vocal cords ___________ from the overuse of voice.

❺ Parkinson's disease is a ___________ disorder of the central nervous system due to the death of dopamine-generating cells in the substantia nigra of the brain.

❻ She fell off her bike and ___________ her knee.

❼ Ten thousand steps a day may keep the ___________ away.

❽ The first sign of Tourette's syndrome is often a ___________, such as eye blinking.

36
지혈대를 매는 방법을 아세요?
Do you know how to apply a tourniquet?

Vocabulary Preview 다음 단어의 뜻을 적어보세요.

❶ amnesia	________	⓰ hypertension	________
❷ bleeding	________	⓱ immune system	________
❸ blister	________	⓲ limb	________
❹ blood flow	________	⓳ loosen	________
❺ blood pressure	________	⓴ memory loss	________
❻ boost	________	㉑ numb	________
❼ cholecystectomy	________	㉒ persistently	________
❽ cold sore	________	㉓ removal	________
❾ convulsion	________	㉔ sneezing	________
❿ deep breathing	________	㉕ stroke	________
⓫ elevated	________	㉖ surgical	________
⓬ esophagitis	________	㉗ take a bath	________
⓭ esophagus	________	㉘ take care of	________
⓮ gallbladder	________	㉙ tourniquet	________
⓯ hiccup	________	㉚ ulcer	________

Short Conversation

A: Excuse me. Can you help me?
실례합니다. 좀 도와줄 수 있나요?

B: What can I do for you?
어떻게 도와드릴까요?

A: **Do you know how to apply a tourniquet?**
지혈대를 매는 방법을 아세요?

B: Oh, you're bleeding. I think I can help stop the bleeding.
오, 피를 흘리시네요. 지혈하는 걸 도와드릴게요.

Pattern Practice

1 Do you know how + to 부정사

1. Do you know how to cure hiccups?
2. Do you know how to stop the bleeding?
3. Do you know how to brush your teeth well?
4. Do you know how to do this exercise correctly?
5. Do you know how to take care of your teeth and gums?

2 Do you know that + 문장

1. Do you know that eggs are good for your brain?
2. Do you know that you have more than 200 bones?
3. Do you know that sneezing helps keep your body safe?
4. Do you know that deep breathing is good for your brain?
5. Do you know that you can boost your immune system by taking a bath?

Useful Expressions

1. We use a tourniquet to control bleeding.
   출혈을 막으려고 지혈대를 사용해요.

2. Tourniquets are tight bands.
   지혈대는 단단히 조이는 밴드예요.

3. Tourniquets are useful in cases of severe bleeding.
   지혈대는 심한 출혈의 경우에 유용해요.

4. Wrap the tourniquet material around the limb several times.
   지혈대 천을 팔이나 다리 둘레에 여러 번 휘감으세요.

5. Make sure that the tourniquet does not loosen.
   지혈대가 느슨하게 풀어지지 않도록 하세요.

Vocabulary Review 박스 안의 적당한 단어를 사용하여 빈칸을 채워보세요.

a. brain	b. convulsions	c. gallbladder	d. hypertension	e. limb
f. memory	g. mouth	h. numb	i. stomach	

❶ A person suffers from ___________ when their blood pressure is persistently elevated beyond a normal level.

❷ Amnesia is a term used to describe full or partial ___________ loss.

❸ Cholecystectomy is the surgical removal of the ___________.

❹ Cold sores are small, blister-like ulcers that occur in and around the ___________.

❺ Esophagitis frequently occurs when acid-containing fluid flows from the ___________ back into the esophagus.

❻ I hate cold weather. Even with gloves, my fingers get ___________.

❼ If blood flow to part of your ___________ stops, a stroke occurs.

❽ She could not drive because she sometimes had ___________.

37
어디가 불편하신가요?
What seems to be the problem?

Vocabulary Preview 다음 단어의 뜻을 적어보세요.

❶ acid reflux ______	⑯ infected ______
❷ AIDS ______	⑰ laboratory test ______
❸ amnesia ______	⑱ mucus ______
❹ Band-Aid ______	⑲ notice ______
❺ blister ______	⑳ overeating ______
❻ blood transfusion ______	㉑ paper cut ______
❼ contact ______	㉒ saliva ______
❽ container ______	㉓ secrete ______
❾ disease ______	㉔ specimen ______
❿ enamel ______	㉕ spread ______
⓫ feces ______	㉖ stomach acid ______
⓬ flow into ______	㉗ stool ______
⓭ gargling ______	㉘ urine ______
⓮ GERD ______	㉙ vital signs ______
⓯ heartburn ______	㉚ wear away ______

Short Conversation

A: What seems to be the problem?
어디가 불편하신가요?

B: I have frequent heartburn.
저는 자주 속이 쓰려요.

A: How long have you had your symptom?
그 증상을 느낀 지 얼마나 오래 되었나요?

B: I have had it all week.
일주일 내내 쓰렸어요.

Pattern Practice

1 What seems to + 동사 원형

1. What seems to be wrong?
2. What seems to be happening?
3. What seems to be the matter?
4. What seems to be the trouble?
5. What seems to be the difficulty?

2 You seem to + 동사 원형

1. You seem to eat too much.
2. You seem to be in great shape.
3. You seem to be in a good mood.
4. You seem to be down this morning.
5. You seem to have gained some weight.

Useful Expressions

1. When did you first notice the pain?
언제부터 통증을 알게 되었어요?

2. I think you need to take some laboratory tests.
임상병리검사를 좀 해봐야겠어요.

3. You need to give a specimen of your urine, stool and blood.
소변과 대변, 그리고 혈액 검사용 시료를 내셔야 합니다.

4. Give the patient a container so we can get a urine specimen.
소변을 받아올 수 있도록 그 환자에게 용기를 주세요.

5. Let me check your vital signs.
맥박과 호흡, 체온, 그리고 혈압을 체크해보겠습니다.

Vocabulary Review 박스 안의 적당한 단어를 사용하여 빈칸을 채워보세요.

a. amnesia	b. aspirin	c. Band-Aids	d. contact	e. gargling
f. infected	g. mouth	h. overeating	i. weight	

❶ Gastroesophageal reflux disease (GERD), acid reflux and heartburn can cause stomach acid to flow into your __________, wearing away the enamel of your teeth.

❷ Hand-foot-and-mouth disease spreads through __________ with saliva, feces, fluid secreted from blisters or mucus from the nose and throat.

❸ He had a stomachache from __________ and ran to the toilet.

❹ He has a headache. He should take some __________.

❺ I just got a paper cut! Do we have any __________?

❻ She got __________ with AIDS during a blood transfusion.

❼ The accident victim has __________ and can't remember her name.

❽ Try __________ with some salt water. It will help your throat.

38
당신은 얼마동안 입원하신 거예요?
How long have you been hospitalized?

Vocabulary Preview 다음 단어의 뜻을 적어보세요.

❶ acne ________	⓰ hearing loss ________
❷ attending doctor ________	⓱ hospitalized ________
❸ Bell's palsy ________	⓲ injury ________
❹ bitter ________	⓳ inpatient ________
❺ combination ________	⓴ lift up ________
❻ contagious ________	㉑ muscle ________
❼ cure ________	㉒ mutation ________
❽ deaf-blindness ________	㉓ on-call ________
❾ dentist ________	㉔ paralysis ________
❿ discharge ________	㉕ reluctant ________
⓫ ease ________	㉖ stab wound ________
⓬ emergency ward ________	㉗ surgical resident ________
⓭ examine ________	㉘ treatment ________
⓮ gene ________	㉙ Usher syndrome ________
⓯ genetic disorder ________	㉚ visual impairment ________

Short Conversation

A: How's your injury? Are you OK?
부상은 어때요? 괜찮아요?

B: I'm feeling better.
좀 나아졌어요.

A: **How long have you been hospitalized?**
당신은 얼마동안 입원하신 거예요?

B: For about two weeks.
2주 정도 되었어요.

Pattern Practice

1 Would you please + 동사 원형

1. Would you please come this way?
2. Would you please call a doctor for me?
3. Would you please show me your ID card?
4. Would you please tell me where the bathroom is?
5. Would you please lift up your shirt? I'll examine you.

2 Why don't you + 동사 원형

1. Why don't you go see a doctor?
2. Why don’t you take some aspirin?
3. Why don't you go home early and get some rest?
4. Why don't you get proper treatment for your acne?
5. Why don't you have milk and yoghurt for your bones?

Useful Expressions

1. Would you please page the surgical resident?
   외과 레지던트를 호출해주시겠습니까?

2. Paging, paging surgical resident Mr. Brian Smith!
   사람을 찾습니다. 외과 레지던트 브라이언 스미스 선생님!

3. Who is today's on-call doctor for the emergency ward?
   오늘의 응급병동 (호출대기) 당직의사는 누구예요?

4. Who is your attending doctor?
   당신의 주치의는 누구예요?

5. The doctor is reluctant to discharge the long-time inpatient.
   의사는 그 장기입원환자를 퇴원시키기를 꺼려요.

Vocabulary Review 박스 안의 적당한 단어를 사용하여 빈칸을 채워보세요.

a. bones	b. contagious	c. cure	d. ease	e. face
f. hearing	g. hospitalized	h. sweet	i. toothache	

❶ He was ___________ with stab wounds.

❷ If your muscle weakness or paralysis affects only your ___________, a more likely cause is Bell's palsy.

❸ I've got a terrible ___________ and I must see the dentist.

❹ Medicine is bitter for the tongue, but ___________ for the body.

❺ The best ___________ for a cold is to rest.

❻ The common cold is a ___________ disease.

❼ These pills will help to ___________ the pain.

❽ Usher syndrome is a relatively rare genetic disorder caused by a mutation in any one of 10 genes resulting in a combination of ___________ loss and visual impairment, and is a leading cause of deaf-blindness.

39

대장암 가족력이 있습니까?

Do you have a family history of colon cancer?

Vocabulary Preview 다음 단어의 뜻을 적어보세요.

❶ anemia ________	⑯ fiber ________
❷ biopsy ________	⑰ hoarse ________
❸ bleeding ________	⑱ loop ________
❹ bowel movement ________	⑲ podiatrist ________
❺ cauterize ________	⑳ prescription ________
❻ chapped ________	㉑ rectum ________
❼ chapstick ________	㉒ screening ________
❽ colon cancer ________	㉓ sigmoidoscopy ________
❾ colon polyp ________	㉔ snoring ________
❿ colonoscopy ________	㉕ stalk ________
⓫ constipation ________	㉖ tarry stool ________
⓬ cramping ________	㉗ thunderous ________
⓭ diabetic ________	㉘ tiredness ________
⓮ endoscope ________	㉙ waistline ________
⓯ facelift ________	㉚ wear off ________

Short Conversation

A: Do you have a family history of colon cancer?
대장암 가족력이 있습니까?

B: No, I don't. Is there anything wrong with my intestines?
아니요, 없습니다. 제 장에 뭔가 이상이 있나요?

A: Polyps were found in your large intestine during the screening colonoscopy, but they were removed completely.
대장내시경 검사에서 대장에 용종이 발견되었는데,
완전히 제거 했습니다.

B: Thank you. How often should I have a colonoscopy?
감사합니다. 대장내시경 검사를 얼마나 자주 해야 하나요?

Pattern Practice

1 Let me + 동사 원형

1. Let me look at your knees.
2. Let me write out the prescription.
3. Let me know when the pain has worn off.
4. Let me wish you a speedy return to health.
5. Let me tell you what you should eat for your heart.

2 I'd like to + 동사 원형

1. I'd like to get a total facelift.
2. I'd like to take you to the doctor's office.
3. I'd like to save the lives of other diabetics.
4. I'd like to make an appointment with Dr. Kim.
5. I'd like to see a doctor as quickly as possible.

Useful Expressions

1. I'd like to take a stomach biopsy.
   위장 조직검사를 받고 싶어요.

2. Let me take a biopsy of the colon.
   대장 조직검사 좀 해주세요.

3. When was your last bowel movement?
   언제 마지막 변을 보셨어요?

4. Do you have a personal history of colon polyps?
   대장용종의 전력이 있습니까?

5. The doctor snaked an endoscope down my throat.
   의사가 나의 목구멍으로 내시경을 요령껏 밀어 넣었어요.

Vocabulary Review 박스 안의 적당한 단어를 사용하여 빈칸을 채워보세요.

a. bleeding	b. constipation	c. foot	d. heart	e. hoarse
f. lips	g. rectum	h. snoring	i. waistline	

❶ Colon cancer can affect the body by causing anemia, tiredness, black or tarry stool and blood in the ___________.

❷ Colon polyps can be removed during a colonoscopy or sigmoidoscopy using a wire loop that cuts the stalk of the polyp and cauterizes it to prevent ___________.

❸ Fiber in the diet promotes regular bowel movements and helps avoid __________ and cramping.

❹ I have a frog in my throat. I mean I have a ___________ throat.

❺ I have gained weight. I think I'll have to reduce my ___________.

❻ I need a chapstick. My ___________ are chapped because of the dry weather.

❼ Podiatrist is the fancy name for a ___________ doctor.

❽ Your thunderous ___________ is really hard to take.

40
당신은 A형 간염에 대한 항체가 없어요.
You don't have an antibody for hepatitis A.

Vocabulary Preview 다음 단어의 뜻을 적어보세요.

❶ abdomen ____________

❷ antibody ____________

❸ appetite ____________

❹ cold sore ____________

❺ contact lens ____________

❻ cough ____________

❼ dry eye ____________

❽ evaporation ____________

❾ gastroscopy ____________

❿ hepatitis ____________

⓫ hypotonia ____________

⓬ illness ____________

⓭ incision ____________

⓮ laparoscopy ____________

⓯ muscle ____________

⓰ obsess ____________

⓱ operation ____________

⓲ ophthalmologist ____________

⓳ osteoarthritis ____________

⓴ pelvis ____________

㉑ predisposition ____________

㉒ prevention ____________

㉓ scoliosis ____________

㉔ sneeze ____________

㉕ spine ____________

㉖ thigh ____________

㉗ tummy ____________

㉘ vaccinate ____________

㉙ vaccination ____________

㉚ wobbly ____________

Short Conversation

A: Are you vaccinated against hepatitis?
간염예방접종 받으셨어요?

B: No, I'm not. I think I need to get a vaccination.
아니요, 받지 않았어요. 저는 예방접종을 받아야 할 것 같아요.

A: Yes, you should.
네, 받으셔야 해요.
You don't have an antibody for hepatitis A.
당신은 A형 간염에 대한 항체가 없어요.

B: OK. I'll get vaccinated right away.
예, 바로 예방접종 받겠습니다.

Pattern Practice

1 You don't have + 명사

1. You don't have a fever.
2. You don't have an appetite.
3. You don't have an acne problem.
4. You don't have any weight to lose.
5. You don't have any wrinkles on your face.

2 You don't have to + 동사 원형

1. You don't have to go to the dentist anymore.
2. You don't have to deal with your illness alone.
3. You don't have to obsess about your diet, but eat healthily.
4. You don't have to worry about your wobbly tummy or thighs.
5. You don't have to go to an ophthalmologist for contact lenses.

Useful Expressions

1. I need to get a vaccination.
   저는 예방접종을 받아야 해요.

2. I have a cold sore.
   저는 입술이 부르터요.

3. I have a cold sore in my mouth.
   저는 입안이 헐어요.

4. It will take a while to heal.
   치유되려면 시간이 꽤 걸려요.

5. I have dry eyes.
   저는 안구건조증이 있어요.

Vocabulary Review 박스 안의 적당한 단어를 사용하여 빈칸을 채워보세요.

a. appetite	b. evaporation	c. face	d. illnesses	e. incisions
f. knee	g. mouth	h. spine	i. stomach	

❶ Accurate knowledge of a patient's family history may identify a predisposition to developing certain ____________, which can inform clinical decisions and allow effective management or even prevention of conditions.

❷ Cover your __________ when you cough or sneeze.

❸ Dry eye syndrome is another eye disease caused by either decreased tear production or increased tear film __________.

❹ Laparoscopy is an operation performed in the abdomen or pelvis through small __________ with the aid of a camera.

❺ Scoliosis generally affects the __________ and hypotonia affects the muscles.

❻ She has completely lost her __________ since the operation.

❼ The most common cause of __________ problems is osteoarthritis.

❽ Your __________ must be empty before gastroscopy.

41
나는 무릎관절에 문제가 있어요.
I have a problem in my knee joints.

Vocabulary Preview 다음 단어의 뜻을 적어보세요.

1. acupoint ________
2. acupuncture ________
3. anesthetic drug ________
4. arthritis ________
5. bleeding ________
6. clean out ________
7. colon ________
8. colonoscopy ________
9. come down with ________
10. consciousness ________
11. esophagus ________
12. gain weight ________
13. high blood pressure ________
14. hypertension ________
15. hypotension ________
16. indigestion ________
17. knee joint ________
18. lose weight ________
19. low blood pressure ________
20. low-key ________
21. melena ________
22. needle-phobic ________
23. neuralgia ________
24. small intestine ________
25. sprain ________
26. stimulation ________
27. stool ________
28. tarry ________
29. wear off ________
30. work out ________

Short Conversation

A: Why are you limping like that?
왜 그렇게 다리를 절룩거리세요?

B: **I have a problem in my knee joints.**
나는 무릎관절에 문제가 있어요.

A: Do you have osteoarthritis?
골관절염이 있으세요?

B: Yes. I should get rid of fluid occasionally because it builds up around my left knee.
예, 제 왼쪽 무릎 주변에 물이 차서 가끔 물을 빼주어야 해요.

Pattern Practice

1 I think + 문장

1. I think you caught a cold
2. I think I've gained some weight.
3. I think I came down with a cold
4. I think I'm suffering from indigestion.
5. I think I sprained my ankle playing soccer.

2 I should + 동사 원형

1. I should go to the hospital.
2. I should take these pills every day.
3. I should keep low-key with food for a while.
4. I should be regularly screened for low blood pressure.
5. I should start working out. I've gained some weight.

Useful Expressions

1. Arthritis involves a lot of pain.
   관절염은 많은 통증을 수반해요.

2. I have severe neuralgia.
   저는 신경통이 심해요.

3. I think I'm coming down with something.
   저는 감기기운이 좀 있는 것 같아요.

4. Get some acupuncture treatment.
   침을 맞아보세요.

5. I'm extremely needle-phobic.
   저는 주사나 침을 무척 무서워해요.

Vocabulary Review 박스 안의 적당한 단어를 사용하여 빈칸을 채워보세요.

a. cleaned out	b. consciousness	c. gain	d. hypertension	e. indigestion
f. lose	g. medicine	h. needles	i. stool	

❶ Acupuncture is the stimulation of specific acupoints along the skin of the body using thin ___________.

❷ As the anesthetic drugs wear off, your ___________ starts to return.

❸ Before colonoscopy, your colon must be completely ___________.

❹ Bleeding that takes place in the esophagus, stomach, or the first part of the small intestine most often causes the ___________ to appear black or tarry. Your doctor may use the term "melena."

❺ Don't eat too much, or you'll have an attack of ___________.

❻ Hypotension is the opposite of ___________, which is high blood pressure.

❼ I caught a cold. Would you prepare some ___________ for me?

❽ If you want to ___________ weight, eat like a bird.

42
나는 매년 독감예방접종을 받아요.
I get a flu shot every year.

Vocabulary Preview 다음 단어의 뜻을 적어보세요.

❶ acute ______________
❷ aftercare ______________
❸ aggravate ______________
❹ allergic rhinitis ______________
❺ breathe in ______________
❻ cervical cancer ______________
❼ clog up ______________
❽ convalescent ______________
❾ cough tablet ______________
❿ crutch ______________
⓫ diphtheria ______________
⓬ head cold ______________
⓭ hematochezia ______________
⓮ indication ______________
⓯ lozenge ______________
⓰ migraine headache ______________
⓱ mucous membrane ______________
⓲ nasal spray ______________
⓳ orthodontist ______________
⓴ pharmacist ______________
㉑ pharyngitis ______________
㉒ physical checkup ______________
㉓ pollen ______________
㉔ prescription ______________
㉕ runny ______________
㉖ sneeze ______________
㉗ sore throat ______________
㉘ stool ______________
㉙ trauma ______________
㉚ treatment ______________

Short Conversation

A: I think I'm coming down with the flu.
나는 독감 기운이 있는 것 같아요.

B: Did you get a flu shot?
독감예방접종 받았어요?

A: No, I didn't. I hate needles, you know.
아니요, 받지 않았어요. 나는 주사 맞는 거 정말 싫어요.

B: It's better safe than sorry.
나중에 걸리고 후회하는 것 보다 미리 조심하는 것이 낫죠.
I get a flu shot every year.
나는 매년 독감예방접종을 받아요.

Pattern Practice

1 I need to + 동사 원형

1. I need to get my prescription filled.
2. I need to take better care of my eyes
3. I need to lose weight and build muscle.
4. I need to use these crutches for six to eight weeks.
5. I need to reschedule my appointment with the orthodontist tomorrow.

2 I want to + 동사 원형

1. I want to lose weight.
2. I want to be a pharmacist.
3. I want to get a physical checkup every year.
4. I want to become a doctor and go into medicine.
5. I want to exercise more and live a healthier lifestyle.

Useful Expressions

1. I have allergic rhinitis.
   나는 알레르기성 비염이 있어요.

2. My nose clogs up when I breathe in something I'm allergic to.
   내가 알레르기를 느끼는 성분을 숨으로 들이마시면 코가 막혀요.

3. I need to use nasal sprays.
   나는 비염 스프레이를 사용해야겠어요.

4. She got a cervical cancer shot last month.
   그녀는 지난달에 자궁경부암 예방주사를 맞았어요.

5. I have a migraine headache from a head cold.
   나는 코감기 때문에 편두통이 있어요.

Vocabulary Review 박스 안의 적당한 단어를 사용하여 빈칸을 채워보세요.

a. blood	b. convalescent	c. indication	d. lozenge	e. muscle
f. pharyngitis	g. result	h. runny	i. sneeze	

❶ A sore throat is usually caused by acute ____________, although it can also appear as a __________ of trauma, diphtheria, or other conditions.

❷ Aftercare is the care and treatment of a __________ patient.

❸ Cough tablets have taken the name _____________, based on their original shape, a diamond.

❹ Hematochezia is the medical term for the presence of 'fresh' ___________ in the stool. Red strands or streaks in the stool or red to pink staining of the toilet bowl water may also be an __________ of hematochezia.

❺ His nose is __________ because he has a cold.

❻ People with allergic rhinitis often __________ outdoors because the pollen in the air aggravates the mucous membrane in the nose.

43
저는 어지러워서 방이 빙빙 돌아가네요.
I feel dizzy, and the room is spinning.

Vocabulary Preview 다음 단어의 뜻을 적어보세요.

❶ acupuncture ________
❷ acute ________
❸ alternative medicine ________
❹ anemia ________
❺ blood flow ________
❻ blood pressure ________
❼ body weight ________
❽ CBC ________
❾ chronic ________
❿ cupping therapy ________
⓫ dizzy ________
⓬ ECG ________
⓭ hemoglobin ________
⓮ hypodermic needle ________
⓯ injection ________
⓰ laboratory slip ________
⓱ measure ________
⓲ mobilize ________
⓳ moxa ________
⓴ moxibustion ________
㉑ mugwart ________
㉒ needle phobia ________
㉓ pale ________
㉔ practitioner ________
㉕ pulse rate ________
㉖ spinning ________
㉗ suction ________
㉘ temperature ________
㉙ vital signs ________
㉚ ward ________

Short Conversation

A: You look so pale. Are you OK?
안색이 좋지 않아요. 괜찮아요?

B: **I feel dizzy, and the room is spinning.**
저는 어지러워서 방이 빙빙 돌아가네요.

A: Do you have anemia?
빈혈 있으세요?

B: No, not that I know of.
아니요, 그렇지는 않아요.
I just didn't get enough sleep last night.
어젯밤에 잠을 충분히 못자서 그래요.

Pattern Practice

1 Let me + 동사 원형

1. Let me feel your forehead.
2. Let me check your vital signs.
3. Let me take your temperature.
4. Let me take you to the hospital.
5. Let me tell you what you should eat for your liver.

2 I have no + 복수 명사

1. I'll change bed sheets.
2. I'll check your body weight.
3. I'll check your blood pressure.
4. I'll give you a tour of this ward.
5. I'll read your weight and measure your height.

Useful Expressions

1. Here's your laboratory slip.
   당신의 임상병리검사 기록용지가 여기 있어요.

2. Let me see the CBC on the laboratory slip.
   임상병리검사 기록용지에 있는 전체 혈구 계산치 내역을 보여주세요.

3. CBC stands for Complete Blood Count.
   CBC는 Complete Blood Count의 약어예요.

4. You need to take an ECG test. ECG stands for electrocardiograph.
   당신은 심전도검사를 받아야 해요. ECG는 electrocardiograph의 약어예요.

5. Please measure my pulse rate.
   저의 맥박횟수를 측정하세요.

Vocabulary Review 박스 안의 적당한 단어를 사용하여 빈칸을 채워보세요.

a. blood flow	b. chronic	c. conditions	d. dizzy	e. fear
f. hemoglobin	g. injections	h. mugwort	i. suction	

❶ Cupping therapy is an ancient Chinese form of alternative medicine in which a local ___________ is created on the skin; practitioners believe this mobilizes ___________ in order to promote healing.

❷ Moxibustion is a traditional Chinese medicine therapy using moxa made from dried ___________.

❸ Needle phobia is the extreme ___________ of medical procedures involving ___________ or hypodermic needles.

❹ Traditionally, acupuncture was used to treat acute _________ while moxibustion was used for ___________ diseases.

❺ When the ___________ levels are lower than normal, blood is less red in color.

44
환자의 침대를 다른 곳으로 옮기려고 하세요?
Are you going to move the patient's gurney to another place?

Vocabulary Preview 다음 단어의 뜻을 적어보세요.

❶ abdominal cavity ______	⑯ I.V. line ______
❷ appendicitis ______	⑰ infectious ______
❸ appendix ______	⑱ larynx ______
❹ biopsy ______	⑲ nutrition ______
❺ blepharoplasty ______	⑳ perforate ______
❻ bronchi ______	㉑ pull loose ______
❼ clutter ______	㉒ removal ______
❽ comatose ______	㉓ respirator ______
❾ cough up ______	㉔ sneeze ______
❿ disconnect ______	㉕ sputum ______
⓫ excess skin ______	㉖ sunscreen ______
⓬ eyelid ______	㉗ surgery ______
⓭ fasten ______	㉘ trachea ______
⓮ gurney ______	㉙ tubing ______
⓯ hemoptysis ______	㉚ tumor ______

Short Conversation

A: Are you going to move the patient's gurney to another place?
환자의 침대를 다른 곳으로 옮기려고 하세요?

B: Yes, I am. Can you help me?
예, 좀 도와주시겠어요?

A: OK. How can I help you? Just let me know.
예, 어떻게 도와드릴까요? 말씀만 하세요.

B: Can you guide a clutter of I.V. lines and other tubing?
침대에 얼기설기 매달린 링거주사용 수액관로를 비롯한
여러 관로들을 좀 유도해주시겠어요?

Pattern Practice

1 Make sure (that) + 문장

1. Make sure you fasten your seatbelt.
2. Make sure you get the right nutrition.
3. Make sure you get a good night's sleep.
4. Make sure you take these drugs on a full stomach.
5. Make sure you brush your teeth before going to bed.

2 Make sure to + 동사 원형

1. Make sure to get enough sleep for your health.
2. Make sure to cover your mouth when you sneeze.
3. Make sure to eat a healthy breakfast every morning.
4. Make sure to wear sunscreen before you go outside.
5. Make sure to wash your hands before eating something.

Useful Expressions

1. The patient is lying comatose on a respirator.
그 환자는 인공호흡기에 매달려 혼수상태로 누워있어요.

2. There's no coworker available to guide a clutter of I.V. lines and other tubing right now.
침대에 얼기설기 매달린 링거주사용 수액관로를 비롯한 여러 관로들을 유도해줄 만한 협력자가 지금 없어요.

3. Move I.V. lines and other tubing first.
링거주사용 수액관로와 여러 연결 관로들을 먼저 이동하세요.

4. Make sure they are out of the way and not in danger of pulling loose.
그것들이 통행에 방해가 되지도 않으면서 잡아당겨 풀어질 위험에 처하지도 않게 하세요.

5. Disconnect tubes from the bed if possible.
연결 관로들은 가능하면 침대에서 분리시키세요.

Vocabulary Review 박스 안의 적당한 단어를 사용하여 빈칸을 채워보세요.

a. biopsy	b. blood	c. burst	d. eyelid	e. removal
f. remove	g. sputum	h. tumor	i. wash	

❶ Appendicitis is a medical emergency that requires prompt surgery to ________ the appendix. Left untreated, an inflamed appendix will eventually __________, or perforate, spilling infectious materials into the abdominal cavity.

❷ Blepharoplasty involves the __________ of excess skin and tightening of the remaining skin on the __________.

❸ Hemoptysis is the act of coughing up __________ or blood-stained ________ from the bronchi, larynx, trachea, or lungs.

❹ If a ________ was found in a routine medical checkup, your doctor will probably want to do a __________ to see if cancer is present.

45
단순한 접촉사고였어요.
It was only a fender-bender.

Vocabulary Preview 다음 단어의 뜻을 적어보세요.

❶ acute shortage	________	⓰ paramedic	________
❷ anxiety disorder	________	⓱ pharmacist	________
❸ bone marrow	________	⓲ PTSD	________
❹ broadside	________	⓳ rear-end	________
❺ coma	________	⓴ recovery	________
❻ damage	________	㉑ resuscitate	________
❼ dieting	________	㉒ self-esteem	________
❽ fender-bender	________	㉓ sideswipe	________
❾ go through	________	㉔ southbound	________
❿ headbanging	________	㉕ surgery	________
⓫ injury	________	㉖ surplus fat	________
⓬ medical attention	________	㉗ sustain	________
⓭ miracle cure	________	㉘ threat	________
⓮ on call	________	㉙ trauma	________
⓯ overweight	________	㉚ whiplash	________

Short Conversation

A: I heard you had a car accident.
당신이 교통사고 났다고 들었어요.

B: Yes, but I'm OK. **It was only a fender-bender.**
예, 그런데 괜찮아요. **단순한 접촉사고였어요.**

A: What a relief! What happened?
정말 다행이에요! 어떻게 사고가 난 거예요?

B: I was rear-ended at a stop light.
정지신호에서 뒤를 받쳤어요.

Pattern Practice

1 There is + 단수 명사(가산/불가산)

1. There is surplus fat in his body.
2. There is a doctor on call 24 hours a day.
3. There is an acute shortage of pharmacists.
4. There is an uncomfortable feeling in my throat.
5. There is still a ray of hope for his recovery.

2 There are + 복수 명사

1. There are no miracle cures involved in dieting.
2. There are large numbers of overweight students.
3. There are many people who don't like to exercise.
4. There are two types of bone marrow—yellow and red.
5. There are countless patients leaving the hospital with higher self-esteem than before the surgery.

Useful Expressions

1. There's an auto accident at km marker 80 on the southbound Gyeongbu Expressway.
경부고속도로 하행선 80km 지점에 교통사고가 났어요.

2. Your first step after an auto accident is to seek and receive immediate medical attention.
교통사고 후 첫째 단계는 즉각적인 의료구조를 받는 것이에요.

3. That Mercedes sideswiped mine.
저 벤츠가 내차 옆을 긁고 지나갔어요.

4. This truck rear-ended my Beemer.
이 트럭이 내 BMW를 추돌했어요.

5. Your car broadsided mine.
당신의 차가 내차의 측면을 받았어요.

Vocabulary Review 박스 안의 적당한 단어를 사용하여 빈칸을 채워보세요.

a. anxiety	b. coma	c. fender-bender	d. injured	e. rear
f. rear-ended	g. resuscitate	h. sustained	i. trauma	

❶ It was just a ______________. I put on my brakes and got tapped by the car behind me. We weren't going fast, so no one was ______________, and there wasn't much damage to either car.

❷ PTSD is a type of ______________ disorder. It can occur after you have gone through an extreme emotional _____________ that involved the threat of injury or death.

❸ The paramedics were unable to ___________ him because he was in a ___________ by the time they arrived.

❹ Whiplash is commonly associated with motor vehicle accidents, usually when the vehicle has been hit in the _________; however, the injury can be ________ in many other ways, including headbanging, bungee jumping and falls.

Answer Key

Vocabulary Review 01

❶ After an <u>operation</u>, another serious inflammation recurred in his left knee.
❷ He needs more time to <u>recuperate</u> from his injury.
❸ He regularly gets checked for metastasis or a <u>recurrence</u> twice a year.
❹ I felt very <u>dizzy</u> all of a sudden and collapsed.
❺ <u>Midwives</u> play a crucial role in supporting normal birth.
❻ Take one <u>pill</u> three times a day.
❼ The blood is chronically short of red blood cells, a condition called <u>anemia</u>.
❽ The cancer tsar himself admits that we have a <u>shortage</u> of radiotherapy capacity in this country.
❾ The <u>surgeon</u> operated on my broken leg last week.
❿ Your <u>family doctor</u> can diagnose and prescribe medications for mental health issues.

Vocabulary Review 02

❶ Arthroplasty is when an entire <u>joint</u> is rebuilt or replaced.
❷ He <u>rescued</u> the boy at the risk of his own life.
❸ How did you cure your <u>acne</u>?
❹ I don't want to <u>spread</u> my germs around the office.
❺ In a treatment room, another doctor put his leg in a <u>cast</u>.
❻ Laser <u>surgery</u> is used with the removal of warts.
❼ Many health <u>insurance</u> policies cover ambulance rides for medical emergencies.
❽ She could feel a <u>lump</u> in her breast.
❾ The judoka <u>dislocated</u> his left shoulder during a competition last year.
❿ Use a humidifier to <u>relieve</u> cough and sore throat.

Vocabulary Review 03

❶ Don't eat too fast, or you'll have an attack of <u>indigestion</u>.
❷ He fell on the ice and <u>sprained</u> his wrist.
❸ His eyes were <u>bloodshot</u> from lack of sleep.

❹ I put an ice bag on her forehead to bring down the fever.
❺ I was sick that day and missed the class.
❻ If you are sick or injured, you may take sick leave without pay for up to one year.
❼ I'm overweight, so I really want to lose weight.
❽ My doctor prescribed sleeping pills so I could get some sleep.
❾ She was so sleepy that she had forty winks in the afternoon.
❿ The pharmacist will fill your prescription.

Vocabulary Review 04

❶ Fiber-rich foods help relieve constipation.
❷ Good sleep is the best remedy for fatigue.
❸ He has a hearing disorder, so you need to speak clearly.
❹ Her hemorrhoids make sitting uncomfortable.
❺ I have trouble sleeping at night.
❻ In an emergency, call 911 for an ambulance.
❼ I've got a blister on my hand from a burn.
❽ Shingles is a viral infection that causes a painful rash.
❾ The chain smokers are at high risk for heart disease.
❿ What is the secret for those who successfully lose weight?

Vocabulary Review 05

❶ I thought acupuncture would hurt, but I couldn't even feel the needles.
❷ I'll check your body weight. Please step on the scales.
❸ Let me take your temperature. Please hold the thermometer under your tongue.
❹ Let's get your vital signs--measure your blood pressure and your heart rate.
❺ My father had a massive heart attack then went into a coma. He is now on an artificial respirator.
❻ Take a deep breath and let it out slowly. I'll feel your pulse.
❼ The doctor wrote me a prescription to help lessen my migraine headaches.
❽ The man is signing in at the reception desk of a medical clinic.
❾ You can get your medicine from the pharmacy.
❿ You have to say "excuse me" if you burp.

Vocabulary Review 06

❶ Do you take any medication regularly?
❷ His legs were swollen with dropsy.
❸ I have never been obese, but I was almost always overweight.
❹ I'd like to make an appointment to see Dr. Kim.
❺ Now I feel a cold coming on with frequent sneezes and sniffles.
❻ Now, many young Korean men are choosing cosmetic surgery to improve their looks.
❼ Please give me a urine sample in the cup.
❽ The physician was sued for malpractice after the patient died.
❾ The tiny hospital treats 1,500 people a day and is open nearly around he clock.
❿ You have to fast 12 hours prior to blood test.

Vocabulary Review 07

❶ I always try to avoid things that will affect my health negatively, such as smoking, drinking, and eating junk food.
❷ I have a hard, obstructive phlegm in my throat.
❸ I misused my voice and now I am suffering from laryngitis.
❹ It is hard to swallow food because of my sore throat.
❺ People with contagious diseases are isolated.
❻ Pneumonia is an infection or inflammation of the lungs.
❼ She's two months pregnant, so she often has morning sickness.
❽ Unlike acute bronchitis, chronic bronchitis is an ongoing, serious disease.
❾ When I woke up, my forehead and back were covered in cold sweat.
❿ You had better not pop the pimple. It'll leave a scar.

Vocabulary Review 08

❶ Cells use glucose for energy after it moves into the bloodstream.
❷ Corticosteroids delivered as a nasal spray can reduce inflammation and control symptoms of allergic rhinitis.
❸ He has an allergy to cats that makes her sneeze.
❹ In rare cases, giardia infection may cause a skin rash or hives.
❺ Asthma is a common disease that effects the lungs.
❻ Nausea was a side effect of the medication.
❼ He was hospitalized and given an intravenous drip after suffering dehydration.
❽ My family doctor prescribed a new medicine for my nasal allergy.

❾ The patient was given an <u>anesthetic</u> before surgery.
❿ The presence of pollen in the atmosphere causes <u>hay fever</u> in some people.

Vocabulary Review 09

❶ I exercised for a change, and now I <u>ache</u> all over.
❷ I have a terrible stomachache, I feel like I'm going to <u>die</u>.
❸ I was bitten by a <u>mosquito</u> and I contracted Japanese encephalitis.
❹ Measles can be prevented by <u>immunization</u> at one year of age.
❺ My father has a <u>sore throat</u> and speaks with a rasp.
❻ Pepsin is a digestive enzyme found in <u>gastric</u> juice.
❼ The doctor is listening to a patient's <u>chest</u> with a stethoscope.
❽ Ulcers occur when digestive juices burn a hole in the <u>stomach</u> lining.
❾ You have <u>tested</u> negative for tuberculosis.
❿ You keep hiccuping. I think it'll stop if you drink some <u>water</u>.

Vocabulary Review 10

❶ A healthy diet should help your body <u>resist</u> infection.
❷ Apply the medicine after carefully reading the <u>directions</u>.
❸ Did you know that your body <u>produces</u> vitamin D if you enjoy the sunshine?
❹ Jaundice is often seen in liver disease such as <u>hepatitis</u> or liver cancer.
❺ Migraines usually involve a severe, throbbing pain on one side of the <u>head</u>, plus nausea.
❻ Prevention is better than <u>cure</u>.
❼ The effects of the painkiller wore off, and my tooth began to <u>hurt</u>.
❽ The patient had her prescription <u>filled</u> at the pharmacy.
❾ You can boost your immune system by <u>taking</u> a bath.
❿ Your <u>skin</u> looks really clear and bright. Did you get a facial?

Vocabulary Review 11

❶ Good sleep is the best <u>remedy</u> for fatigue.
❷ I don't feel very well, so I'll take a <u>rest</u> at home.
❸ I got an ultrasonography of my internal organs. I also got an <u>endoscopy</u> of my stomach and my large intestine.
❹ I needed to wear <u>braces</u> to straighten my crooked teeth.
❺ I'm overweight. I want to <u>lose</u> some weight.

❻ It's so itchy that I can't help scratching through my shirt.
❼ My legs feel numb, so I can't walk.
❽ My throat hurts when I swallow something.
❾ Sinusitis occurs when the nasal cavity is blocked and becomes inflamed.
❿ When I blow my nose, my ears squeak.

Vocabulary Review 12

❶ Antibodies found in breast milk protect babies against infection.
❷ Excessive sodium intake can cause health problems.
❸ He put a soothing balm on his cut.
❹ If the ointments do not work, injections or other therapies need to be considered.
❺ Prompt treatment can reduce your risk of complications.
❻ She dropped out of the race because of an injury.
❼ The fatality rate is much higher for patients with chronic liver disease or diabetes.
❽ The symptoms of food poisoning include stomachache, vomiting, and diarrhea.
❾ When a mosquito bites us, that spot gets itchy and swollen.
❿ You have to reposition a patient frequently to prevent bedsores.

Vocabulary Review 13

❶ Aspirin and cold medicine are available over the counter.
❷ Appointments for consultations need to be made at least a day in advance.
❸ He attempted to revive his girl friend who had fainted.
❹ He learned how to do CPR in an emergency when he was ten years old.
❺ He was found lying unconscious on the road.
❻ It is an infectious disease like the flu.
❼ People with diabetes must use this drug regularly.
❽ There were two people injured in the accident.
❾ We are well trained to handle any reasonable emergency.
❿ We called the emergency number and the paramedics were here in no time.

Vocabulary Review 14

❶ Almost two thirds of the fat in avocados is monounsaturated, a type that helps to lower levels of LDL or "bad" cholesterol in the blood.
❷ Are you keeping an eye on your cholesterol level?

❸ Let me give you a shot and <u>prescribe</u> some antibiotics.
❹ The lack of <u>blood flow</u> to your heart during a heart attack leads to irreversible damage to your heart muscle.
❺ The leg was going <u>numb</u> from lack of circulation.
❻ This process is called arteriosclerosis, or <u>hardening</u> of the arteries.
❼ Urinate into the toilet a few seconds before <u>urinating</u> in the sample cup.
❽ When <u>yawning</u>, try not to open your mouth too wide.

Vocabulary Review 15

❶ A few days after giving up smoking, I started to suffer from <u>withdrawal</u> symptoms.
❷ As she has a <u>phobia</u> of water, she doesn't swim.
❸ He had his broken arm in a <u>cast</u> to help the bones knit together.
❹ He is now fighting his <u>addiction</u> to alcohol.
❺ Her cheeks became hollow after several days of <u>sickness</u>.
❻ I went to the <u>dentist</u> and had my teeth scaled.
❼ Monounsaturated and polyunsaturated fats are generally found in <u>plants</u> and are touted as healthy fats, unlike trans fats, saturated fats and cholesterol.
❽ My <u>gums</u> bleed when I brush my teeth.

Vocabulary Review 16

❶ His hands shook as though he had hand <u>tremor</u>.
❷ How many <u>teeth</u> did the dentist take out?
❸ In some people, esophageal <u>spasms</u> can lead to chronic swallowing problems and pain.
❹ Schizophrenia is one of the most common <u>mental</u> illnesses.
❺ She can't <u>drive</u> because she suffers from epilepsy.
❻ She gets <u>claustrophobia</u> in elevators and closets.
❼ Take one pill a day. Do not take an <u>overdose</u>.
❽ The surgeon set her broken arm in <u>splints</u> to hold it in position.

Vocabulary Review 17

❶ During an asthma attack, you may cough, wheeze and have trouble <u>breathing</u>.
❷ I need to <u>draw</u> some blood from you. Make a tight fist, please.
❸ I recommend that you <u>stay away</u> from irritating foods, alcohol and smoking.
❹ I suffer from <u>sciatica</u> so it's hard for me to walk quickly.

❺ If you have frequent attacks of heartburn or indigestion, call your doctor for an appointment.
❻ If you have vertigo it seems as if the room is spinning around you.
❼ Some of the physical symptoms include panic attack, dizziness, trembling, sweating, chest pain, accelerated heart rate, and shortness of breath.
❽ You seem to be very healthy. Do you have any medical problems?

Vocabulary Review 18

❶ After her baby was born, she began cupping therapy to cleanse her body.
❷ Fiber in the diet promotes regular bowel movements and helps avoid constipation and cramping.
❸ Hypertension is one of the most common cardiovascular diseases in Asia, but many people know little or nothing about it.
❹ I burned myself on the stove and got a blister.
❺ I sometimes lose a little bit of hair when I brush my hair.
❻ In his youth, he suffered an attack of Bell's palsy, permanently leaving the left side of his face partially paralyzed.
❼ Insomnia is the most common sleep disorder.
❽ Until a scab forms over the wound, leave it alone.

Vocabulary Review 19

❶ A cold produces such symptoms as a headache, coughing, and a runny nose.
❷ Colon cleansing involves getting rid of the impacted fecal matter found in your intestines.
❸ He is recovering after the surgery for a brain tumor.
❹ I'll give you some medicine for the pain.
❺ It's better to avoid cold food when you have an upset stomach.
❻ She was taken to the hospital with acute appendicitis.
❼ Since the pancreas, surrounded by other organs, is located deep in the abdomen, it is difficult to diagnose pancreatic cancer in its early stage of development.
❽ The level of immunity is bound to drop when the body weakens.

Vocabulary Review 20

❶ He was crippled by polio as a child.
❷ I don't eat any meat. I'm a vegetarian.

❸ I should take this medicine for kidney disease.
❹ She fell off a ladder and broke her arm.
❺ She lost too much blood and passed out.
❻ Snoring may be a symptom of a more serious problem called sleep apnea.
❼ The following medical conditions increase your risk of developing peritonitis: cirrhosis, appendicitis, Crohn's disease, stomach ulcers, diverticulitis and pancreatitis.
❽ Vegetarians usually have lower levels of heart disease.

Vocabulary Review 21

❶ Also called eczema, dermatitis is an inflammation of the skin.
❷ Chocolate is not the cause of tooth decay. The sugar in chocolate can cause cavities.
❸ Gastric bypass is the favored bariatric surgery in the United States.
❹ He had to give himself daily injections of insulin to help him control his blood sugar.
❺ Hearing aids are a common answer for the treatment of tinnitus.
❻ I'm on a diet now. I have to watch what I eat.
❼ In advanced cirrhosis, the liver no longer works.
❽ Saturated fat can contribute to heart disease by increasing levels of bad cholesterol in the blood.

Vocabulary Review 22

❶ A dentist checks and treats your teeth, and a dermatologist is a skin doctor.
❷ Colon cancer and rectal cancer may be associated with a diet low in fiber and high in fat and calories.
❸ He broke his leg and is on crutches now.
❹ He had to give himself daily injections of insulin to help him control his blood sugar.
❺ In my family, we have a history of heart disease and diabetes.
❻ Keeping your scalp clean is vital for hair loss prevention.
❼ Snacking between meals ruins your appetite.
❽ The symptoms of carpal tunnel syndrome start slowly, and you may feel tingling, itching or burning feeling of numbness in fingers and the palms of the hand.

Vocabulary Review 23

❶ After the wound was left untreated, blood poisoning developed.
❷ Chronic fatigue can be alleviated by liver detoxification.

❸ Did you know that your body releases 70 percent of its toxins through breathing?
❹ Heredity also may play a role in the development of salivary gland cancer.
❺ If you have severe bleeding, you could develop anemia.
❻ Leukemia, or cancer of the blood, is the most common type in children.
❼ This medicine will relieve you of your pain.
❽ Vitamins were discovered to correct deficiency diseases such as scurvy, beriberi, and rickets.

Vocabulary Review 24

❶ Dry eye syndrome is another eye disease caused by either decreased tear production or increased tear film evaporation.
❷ Experts recommend using a sunscreen with an SPF of 30 or higher and say it is important to cover every part of your body that will be exposed to the sun.
❸ Gastritis is an inflammation of the lining of the stomach.
❹ My throat is not sore, but I'm a little hoarse from a cold.
❺ Overexposure to ultraviolet rays can cause skin cancer.
❻ While I was suffering from pinkeye, I thought about the hardships of the blind.
❼ Why are your eyes bloodshot? Here, try these eye drops.
❽ Your body has an immune system to fight off germs.

Vocabulary Review 25

❶ Hyperhidrosis is a medical condition, where the body sweats three- to four-times the normal amount.
❷ I can't get rid of the pimples on my face.
❸ I got my wisdom teeth pulled out last year.
❹ Malnutrition is a medical condition, not just a lack of food.
❺ Many of the common childhood diseases such as measles, mumps, chicken pox were mostly eradicated with a national program of vaccinations.
❻ Moxibustion is the application of heat from an herbal bundle, used in conjunction with acupuncture, to stimulate the acupoints on the body and encourage self-healing.
❼ The part bitten by an insect became swollen.
❽ When she was pregnant, she often got morning sickness.

Vocabulary Review 26

❶ Frequent or constant heartburn is the most common symptom of reflux esophagitis.
❷ Ginseng is prescribed alone or in combination with other herbs to treat chronic fatigue, anemia, gastritis, bronchitis, asthma and many other ailments.
❸ If one drinks all his life, he may die of cirrhosis of the liver.
❹ Many women who work on their feet all day suffer from varicose veins and chronic leg and joint problems.
❺ My eyes smart with smoke. Could you put out that cigar?
❻ People with severe panic disorder cannot drive or even step out of the house.
❼ Stretch your arms to get the kinks out of your muscles.
❽ Water is very important during and after a workout to prevent dehydration.

Vocabulary Review 27

❶ Colitis is a chronic digestive disease characterized by inflammation of the colon
❷ Epilepsy is a common chronic neurological disorder characterized by seizures.
❸ I can't chew any food well because of toothache.
❹ I have to get my teeth scaled.
❺ Laughter can speed up recuperation from sickness.
❻ Many doctors say that these artificial sweeteners can boost people's appetites, making them eat more.
❼ The doctor diagnosed her case as tuberculosis.
❽ The surgeon operated on my broken leg last week.

Vocabulary Review 28

❶ Always read the precautions on the bottle before using.
❷ Don't just take pills. Go to a hospital and get a shot.
❸ Don't let it take precedence over your health.
❹ Don't take this product unless directed by a doctor if you have a breathing problem such as emphysema or chronic bronchitis.
❺ He has terminal cancer. With treatment, he may live another year.
❻ If pain persists or gets worse, if new symptoms occur, or if redness or swelling is present, consult a doctor because these could be signs of a serious condition.
❼ My doctor upped my dose because I didn't get better.
❽ Take one pill a day. Do not take an overdose.

Vocabulary Review 29

❶ I can't read books because I can't see the letters. I think I need to wear glasses.
❷ I can't sleep because my roommate is snoring so loudly.
❸ I don't feel very well. Can you recommend a good doctor?
❹ If caffeine keeps you up at night, do not take this product in the evening since it contains natural caffeine.
❺ I'll give you some lidocaine, and then I'll begin working on this filling.
❻ My neck is so stiff that I can't even look back.
❼ Tartar is a hard yellowish substance that forms on your teeth and causes them to decay if it is not removed.
❽ These conditions require immediate care, because if left untreated, seizures and loss of consciousness can occur.

Vocabulary Review 30

❶ Complications that may develop during a coma include pressure sores, bladder infections and pneumonia.
❷ Do you have any aspirin? My head is killing me.
❸ He yawned without covering his mouth.
❹ Smoking is the main cause of chronic bronchitis, which is an incurable disease.
❺ The most common form of dementia is Alzheimer's disease.
❻ Too much intake of ice-cream made me put on fat.
❼ Untreated diabetes can cause dehydration by causing frequent urination.
❽ Using diet pills is not a safe way to lose weight.

Vocabulary Review 31

❶ At the time when the bones are growing, sufficient calcium intake is very important.
❷ Consuming a diet that is high in acid can result in heartburn, stomach pain, and more serious conditions like kidney stones and gout.
❸ If you have severe anemia you may need to be hospitalized and receive blood transfusions.
❹ One type of plastic surgery is rhinoplasty, or nose surgery.
❺ Secondhand smoke is a known risk factor for lung cancer.
❻ The injured were carried away on stretchers.
❼ The nurse was busy taking care of her patients.
❽ You are not allowed to up the dosage without prescription.

Vocabulary Review 32

❶ Her heart had stopped, but the doctors successfully resuscitated her.
❷ I have trouble climbing steps. I have to stop and catch my breath.
❸ Keep the dosage as directed. Overdose may prove harmful.
❹ The patient's lethargy after surgery is normal.
❺ Too much intake of ice cream made me put on fat.
❻ Unable to stand or even sit up, he was hoisted onto a stretcher.
❼ Unless you eat plenty of fruits and vegetables, you may need to take a supplement of vitamin C to achieve the recommended daily dose of 1,000 milligrams.
❽ You have an irregular set of teeth. You need to have braces fixed on your teeth.

Vocabulary Review 33

❶ Cyclothymia is a mild form of bipolar disorder.
❷ He has increasingly shown symptoms of Parkinson's, as shuffling his feet and sometimes grimacing in pain.
❸ I felt her forehead, and she had a fever.
❹ I had some spoiled food and had diarrhea all night.
❺ Septicemia can happen when an infection in the body enters the bloodstream.
❻ She's never been absent before. Maybe she's sick.
❼ Simple motor tics can be explained as eye blinking, nose twitching, and rapid jerking of any part of the body.
❽ What treatments do you recommend for this disorder?

Vocabulary Review 34

❶ An example of a facial tic is mouth twitching or rapidly blinking eyes.
❷ Apply this lotion on your hands. It will soften your skin.
❸ Bell's palsy causes sudden weakness and paralysis in your facial muscles.
❹ Cystitis is the medical term for inflammation of the bladder.
❺ Gently tip his head back so that the Adam's apple is exposed to clear his airways and open his mouth.
❻ It will be all over with your health if you keep on smoking.
❼ You should put on some weight. You look a little too skinny.
❽ You should rest if you're tired.

Vocabulary Review 35

❶ Alopecia is the general medical term for hair loss.
❷ His face is bumpy because of the acne scars.
❸ I have indigestion, and my stomach feels bloated.
❹ I have my vocal cords swollen from the overuse of voice.
❺ Parkinson's disease is a degenerative disorder of the central nervous system due to the death of dopamine-generating cells in the substantia nigra of the brain.
❻ She fell off her bike and bruised her knee.
❼ Ten thousand steps a day may keep the doctor away.
❽ The first sign of Tourette's syndrome is often a facial tic, such as eye blinking.

Vocabulary Review 36

❶ A person suffers from hypertension when their blood pressure is persistently elevated beyond a normal level.
❷ Amnesia is a term used to describe full or partial memory loss.
❸ Cholecystectomy is the surgical removal of the gallbladder.
❹ Cold sores are small, blister-like ulcers that occur in and around the mouth.
❺ Esophagitis frequently occurs when acid-containing fluid flows from the stomach back into the esophagus.
❻ I hate cold weather. Even with gloves, my fingers get numb.
❼ If blood flow to part of your brain stops, a stroke occurs.
❽ She could not drive because she sometimes had convulsions.

Vocabulary Review 37

❶ Gastroesophageal reflux disease (GERD), acid reflux and heartburn can cause stomach acid to flow into your mouth, wearing away the enamel of your teeth.
❷ Hand-foot-and-mouth disease spreads through contact with saliva, feces, fluid secreted from blisters or mucus from the nose and throat.
❸ He had a stomachache from overeating and ran to the toilet.
❹ He has a headache. He should take some aspirin.
❺ I just got a paper cut! Do we have any Band-Aids?
❻ She got infected with AIDS during a blood transfusion.
❼ The accident victim has amnesia and can't remember her name.
❽ Try gargling with some salt water. It will help your throat.

Vocabulary Review 38

❶ He was <u>hospitalized</u> with stab wounds.
❷ If your muscle weakness or paralysis affects only your <u>face</u>, a more likely cause is Bell's palsy.
❸ I've got a terrible <u>toothache</u> and I must see the dentist.
❹ Medicine is bitter for the tongue, but <u>sweet</u> for the body.
❺ The best <u>cure</u> for a cold is to rest.
❻ The common cold is a <u>contagious</u> disease.
❼ These pills will help to <u>ease</u> the pain.
❽ Usher syndrome is a relatively rare genetic disorder caused by a mutation in any one of 10 genes resulting in a combination of <u>hearing</u> loss and visual impairment, and is a leading cause of deaf-blindness.

Vocabulary Review 39

❶ Colon cancer can affect the body by causing anemia, tiredness, black or tarry stool and blood in the <u>rectum</u>.
❷ Colon polyps can be removed during a colonoscopy or sigmoidoscopy using a wire loop that cuts the stalk of the polyp and cauterizes it to prevent <u>bleeding</u>.
❸ Fiber in the diet promotes regular bowel movements and helps avoid <u>constipation</u> and cramping.
❹ I have a frog in my throat. I mean I have a <u>hoarse</u> throat.
❺ I have gained weight. I think I'll have to reduce my <u>waistline</u>.
❻ I need a chapstick. My <u>lips</u> are chapped because of the dry weather.
❼ Podiatrist is the fancy name for a <u>foot</u> doctor.
❽ Your thunderous <u>snoring</u> is really hard to take.

Vocabulary Review 40

❶ Accurate knowledge of a patient's family history may identify a predisposition to developing certain <u>illnesses</u>, which can inform clinical decisions and allow effective management or even prevention of conditions.
❷ Cover your <u>mouth</u> when you cough or sneeze.
❸ Dry eye syndrome is another eye disease caused by either decreased tear production or increased tear film <u>evaporation</u>.
❹ Laparoscopy is an operation performed in the abdomen or pelvis through small <u>incisions</u> with the aid of a camera.

❺ Scoliosis generally affects the spine and hypotonia affects the muscles.
❻ She has completely lost her appetite since the operation.
❼ The most common cause of knee problems is osteoarthritis.
❽ Your stomach must be empty before gastroscopy.

Vocabulary Review 41

❶ Acupuncture is the stimulation of specific acupoints along the skin of the body using thin needles.
❷ As the anesthetic drugs wear off, your consciousness starts to return.
❸ Before colonoscopy, your colon must be completely cleaned out.
❹ Bleeding that takes place in the esophagus, stomach, or the first part of the small intestine most often causes the stool to appear black or tarry. Your doctor may use the term "melena."
❺ Don't eat too much, or you'll have an attack of indigestion.
❻ Hypotension is the opposite of hypertension, which is high blood pressure.
❼ I caught a cold. Would you prepare some medicine for me?
❽ If you want to lose weight, eat like a bird.

Vocabulary Review 42

❶ A sore throat is usually caused by acute pharyngitis, although it can also appear as a result of trauma, diphtheria, or other conditions.
❷ Aftercare is the care and treatment of a convalescent patient.
❸ Cough tablets have taken the name lozenge, based on their original shape, a diamond.
❹ Hematochezia is the medical term for the presence of 'fresh' blood in the stool. Red strands or streaks in the stool or red to pink staining of the toilet bowl water may also be an indication of hematochezia.
❺ His nose is runny because he has a cold.
❻ People with allergic rhinitis often sneeze outdoors because the pollen in the air aggravates the mucous membrane in the nose.

Vocabulary Review 43

❶ Cupping therapy is an ancient Chinese form of alternative medicine in which a local suction is created on the skin; practitioners believe this mobilizes blood flow in order to promote healing.

❷ Moxibustion is a traditional Chinese medicine therapy using moxa made from dried mugwort.
❸ Needle phobia is the extreme fear of medical procedures involving injections or hypodermic needles.
❹ Traditionally, acupuncture was used to treat acute conditions while moxibustion was used for chronic diseases.
❺ When the hemoglobin levels are lower than normal, blood is less red in color.

Vocabulary Review 44

❶ Appendicitis is a medical emergency that requires prompt surgery to remove the appendix. Left untreated, an inflamed appendix will eventually burst, or perforate, spilling infectious materials into the abdominal cavity.
❷ Blepharoplasty involves the removal of excess skin and tightening of the remaining skin on the eyelid.
❸ Hemoptysis is the act of coughing up blood or blood-stained sputum from the bronchi, larynx, trachea, or lungs.
❹ If a tumor was found in a routine medical checkup, your doctor will probably want to do a biopsy to see if cancer is present.

Vocabulary Review 45

❶ It was just a fender-bender. I put on my brakes and got tapped by the car behind me. We weren't going fast, so no one was injured, and there wasn't much damage to either car.
❷ PTSD is a type of anxiety disorder. It can occur after you have gone through an extreme emotional trauma that involved the threat of injury or death.
❸ The paramedics were unable to resuscitate him because he was in a coma by the time they arrived.
❹ Whiplash is commonly associated with motor vehicle accidents, usually when the vehicle has been hit in the rear; however, the injury can be sustained in many other ways, including headbanging, bungee jumping and falls.